BEAUTY
FOR THE
MATURE WOMAN

BEAUTY
FOR THE
MATURE WOMAN

Dorothy Seiffert

Illustrations by Ray Skibinski

HAWTHORN BOOKS, INC.
Publishers / NEW YORK

To my mother, whose example of living
her retiring years with such grace and understanding
inspired this book

BEAUTY FOR THE MATURE WOMAN

Copyright © 1977 by Dorothy Seiffert. Copyright under International and Pan-American Copyright Conventions. All rights reserved, including the right to reproduce this book or portions thereof in any form, except for the inclusion of brief quotations in a review. All inquiries should be addressed to Hawthorn Books, Inc., 260 Madison Avenue, New York, New York 10016. This book was manufactured in the United States of America and published simultaneously in Canada by Prentice-Hall of Canada, Limited, 1870 Birchmount Road, Scarborough, Ontario.

Library of Congress Catalog Card Number: 76-53394

ISBN: 0-8015-3100-4

3 4 5 6 7 8 9 10

Contents

Preface · viii

1
Attitudes to Keep You Young · 3

2
Skin Care · 23

3
Makeup, False Eyelashes and All · 37

4
Diet for the Woman with Too Many Pounds · 55

5
Vitamins to Keep You Healthy · 73

6
Exercise and Stay Young 99

7
Move Like a Teen-ager in 10 Easy Lessons 111

8
Wear Becoming and Fashionable Clothes 121

9
Summing Up 165

Index 177

Preface

My reason for writing this book is to give you a project—*you!* I believe that when our young stop needing us we had better stop needing them and what better way than to find a new interest—*ourselves*. The rewards will be great. Every improvement in this book will bring you more beauty, health, and self-understanding, which adds up to greater pride and self-confidence.

You are going to add to your appearance with a careful selection of clothes. You are going to make yourself more beautiful through skin-care suggestions and correct makeup instructions. You are going to start taking off unnecessary weight with diet and exercise. You are going to build a stronger body with good nutrition, diet supplements, and exercise. You are going to analyze your thinking to search for any negative ruts you may have developed. You are going to expand your life outside your home with helpful projects—helpful to others and to yourself.

I am aware that all of this will take awhile. I recommend working with one chapter at a time so you will retain each improvement before going on to the next. The Rule of Ten structure makes it easy to refer back and forth. Remember that the project is *you* and you are worth both the time and the effort.

Acknowledgments

I would like to thank the following friends who have given me support and assurance in writing this book: Patricia House, Peter Glenn, Sue Long, Ann Seaton, and Beverly Penberthy; Dorothy Brean for her helpful suggestions in the manuscript; Denise Taylor for her help in preparing the vitamin chapter; Elizabeth Backman and Ellane Hoose for their fine eye in editing this book; and last to my son, Stephen Seiffert, and my daughter, Mrs. Susan Maciel, who spurred me on when I faltered.

BEAUTY
FOR THE
MATURE WOMAN

1
Attitudes to Keep You Young

What do you think of *you?* All the rest of you can be together—and you still may not have a healthy attitude toward yourself and others around you. You may have gotten into some ruts of thinking through the years that need to be brought to the surface. If you see in yourself a lack of the following behavior patterns and truthfully find where you stand in each, you may find some improvements that need to be made.

Here is a Rule of Ten for a better-thinking you:

1. Self-Awareness

What is it? My own interpretation is that it is an objective view of your own behavior. I visualize a second person standing aside watching, analyzing, giving advice and criticism. I call him Mr. Right.

Example: I am talking to a friend about her dog. She tells me the dog got in a fight with the dog across the street and got its ear torn.

My first impulse is to tell her about a dog I had once that had his ear torn, too. Mr. Right says to me: She's not interested in your dog right now. She wants sympathy and advice about hers. I comply with Mr. Right.

Self-awareness helps you think and react with intelligence and understanding to what is going on at the moment. It is really to help in your awareness of others. Maybe you think back on a confrontation and say to yourself, "Why did I say that to him?" Mr. Right comes back later to chide you.

Self-awareness is necessary to see your position in a group. Do you enter a roomful of people and verbally control it with the subject that *you* want to talk about? Do you feel uncomfortable with a very young group and consequently try to take over? Just remember that they want to control the thinking of the group themselves. You can be included if you encompass their ideas and try to understand them. If you try to impose your ideas on them, you put yourself in the position of an old fogy. And the group will slowly drift away.

Edmund Burke said, "The arrogance of age must submit to be taught by youth."

How is your self-awareness in your relationship with young people? Can you stand back and see them as adults, or are you still treating them as though they have to be told to wear their mittens?

Do you take the time to find out what makes a child tick? Can you respect an adult child's decision when it is contrary to your own views? Do you stand aside and really see your relationship with children?

Being conscious that my self-awareness might not be working for me all of the time, I tried something recently. I asked my son to tell me when I was doing anything to annoy him or his wife. This may be tricky and I must be prepared to have my feelings hurt. But this seems better to me than having my daughter-in-law possibly say, "I'm always glad when your mother leaves. I never can get into my own kitchen when she is here." Isn't it better to know what you are doing wrong? Disrespect, hurting one's parents' feelings, bears such a taboo that many impossible family relationships develop because the annoyances cannot be expressed.

In your relationship with your in-laws you will need Mr. Right on hand frequently. Stand back and take a look at your position. You are the villain from whom they must lure their spouses. Sweet and dear as they may be, this subconscious problem is there. If you can let them know you are not competing—and don't—you will win their trust and respect.

The grandmother's role is an enviable one. In the majority of families they slip in and out of a child's life, mostly on pleasant occasions. The humdrum daily hassle is left, rightly, to the parents. However, this has its hazards. A person-to-person relationship with a child, especially in a large family, is missing. If you are aware of this and make an effort to develop something special between each one, you will enjoy the role of grandparenthood all the more.

They often say the grandmother's privilege is to spoil the children. It is indeed a privilege if it doesn't go too far, if your self-awareness doesn't help you to see when your indulgence is being frowned upon. "Oh, let him have another piece of cake, it won't hurt him." Everybody laughs but they may not be happy.

Maybe you are too strict with them. Maybe you feel they are running wild and you step in firmly to stop this undisciplined behavior. Where is your self-awareness now? You are imposing your criterion of permissiveness when it is really the parents' decision, isn't it? What permanent change can you bring about by imposing discipline in part-time exposures?

Grandparents must always have their self-awareness with them, for certain. They are in a vulnerable position between parent and child and they must "play it cool."

Your husband: I will only touch lightly on this most complicated relationship of all. Can your newly developed self-awareness help you see the same old daily situations from *his* point of view? Does he really like it if you call him at the office to bring home a loaf of bread? Have you been doing this for so many years that he doesn't even know it is an irritation, until it stops? Try out a few changes that your self-awareness can see might please him. Stand back and look. Your relationship is going into its closest period, according to all the books on retirement. If you live through the first thirty years, you have it made.

How do you get along with the casual relationships in your life? I mean the butcher, the mailman, the waiter. How do you handle yourself in quick brushes with people? Your self-awareness can help you to make pleasant encounters or it can be missing and make you demanding, complaining, and suspicious. Keep Mr. Right with you to remind you that the mailman's feet probably hurt and the waiter may just have had a fight with the cook. Take advice from your new sidekick and show a little sympathy and understanding.

2. Self-Assurance

It is my hope that this book will take you into new areas of pride and self-assurance, areas of your life that you have not paid much attention to; areas of your life that when you expand them will give you a new look at yourself. If you lose a little weight, get a new eye makeup, exercise yourself into a freer movement, add energy to your body with vitamins, or find a new interest, this book will have added to your self-assurance.

Where you get your self-assurance only you can evaluate. I remember one time, during a very low period of self-esteem, I went to a gathering of townspeople in the new community to which I had just moved. When we began to sing my eye was caught by the woman playing the piano because her every body motion and facial expression was full of pride and self-confidence. This simple rural woman had something I didn't. Why? Because she was doing something. I was depressed, because I had no pride in accomplishment in this new place. I soon fixed that by joining everything in sight.

Look for your friends' pride and honor it, because it is the keystone to their self-esteem. I have one friend who spends her all—

both time and money—on her house, another who is rarely home, because she is always out riding her horse.

Psychocybernetics is the study of how one sees one's self, one's self-image. If you think of yourself as a woman who is friendly, outgoing, and loving, you will follow this behavior pattern. If you think yourself ugly, retiring, and stupid, this image will cause you to react negatively to people—and they will respond in kind. Let Mr. Right help you stand back, and look at yourself. What is your self-image? What can this book do to help you build your self-assurance?

3. Keeping Yourself Current

If you want to keep in contact with your peers, with your younger friends, with children, keep yourself informed on their interests and on present-day events.

You will never find yourself at a loss for some conversation beside the weather if you read the newspapers every day. Your self-awareness can help you to choose the subject matter you read with a thought of others' interests as well as your own. It is impossible to be informed on every subject that interests everyone in your life, but the more you know the more easily a common ground can be found.

Sources for widening your horizons lie in books, magazines, some television, travel, seeking out interesting people, going to museums, to name a few. If you choose your books carefully, you always can have something current to talk about. Television has some very informative programs—if you eliminate contest shows. Turn to the educational channels occasionally.

Recently I heard someone remark about a mutual friend: "She might as well have stayed home for all she got out of that trip." When you travel, seek out the places of interest. There are usually pamphlets or books available at most American and foreign historical spots. If you buy these and read them, they can make your trip a lot more valuable to you. Don't go home with only a lot of pictures in your mind, which become a blur after awhile. Looking at the books from time to time you can relive the whole trip. A daily diary is even more fun.

Keeping informed on sports can endear you to all kinds of people. My doorman and I exchange baseball standings, sharing the grief of losing and the joy of winning every day in the season.

Maybe you would enjoy really getting to know about some subject. Take a course, read books, get to be an authority. Great for the ego!

The truth is, the more you know, the more interesting you are. So there!

4. Conversation

I am real hung up on conversation. *The American Heritage Dictionary* defines it as "an informal spoken exchange of thoughts and feelings." The key word is *exchange*—and how frequently it is not the case.

The next time you are with a friend, be sure that Mr. Right is with you. Stand back and be aware of how the conversation proceeds. How many times do you present the subject matter? How many times does your friend? When the subject is established, do you invite comments or do you carry on a monologue that it is impossible to interrupt even with a yes or no? If the subjects are evenly divided between you, do you turn all of hers back to yourself and your opinions, shuffling them right away from her?

Do you jump from one subject to another without a stop for breath? "Joe and I went to the movies but my foot went to sleep. I didn't sleep well the night before, anyway, because the Joneses came over and I drank too much coffee and Margaret talked all evening about her crazy son, not like our Bob who has always been so reliable, you know"—and on and on. The question is, how Margaret could have gotten even a word in edgeways, much less talk all evening.

Do you start each conversation with, "The most awful thing happened," and never introduce a pleasant note in the whole evening? Something terrible is happening to your car; the mayor has no business picking on welfare; Joe's boss is an imbecile; there is nothing decent on television any more; yakety, yakety.

If someone asks you a polite question, such as "How is Aunt Bessie?" do you go on and on? Watch for the set jaw and the glassy eyes as you go through her operation step by step.

Is your only subject of conversation about your children and grandchildren? You'd better watch it, or you will soon be talking to yourself alone.

Do you pounce on every subject, happy with a good stiff argument? Do you put down the other guy whenever possible? Do you take the ball and run with it to show how smart you are—at other people's expense?

Do you and your husband both take on a subject, interrupting one another constantly—two against one? "We got into New York at 6:02." "No, dear, that was Washington at 6:02. We landed at La Guardia at 7:03." Could your victim possibly care?

Whenever anyone heard I was writing a book for older women, without hesitation they said, "Tell them not to repeat themselves." This commonest of all conversation annoyances is not a problem of doddering old age alone. Some of my younger friends are guilty of this, too. Psychiatrists say that this comes from our need to hold onto what we know, to maintain contact with others rather than to accept new thoughts in areas that we can't control.

What to do about it? Mr. Right can help you out if you are constantly aware of what you are saying. There are people who ask, "Have I told you this before?" The answer, of course, is "I don't know." However, if your question is, "Have I told you about the time Joe's horse got loose in the field?" you have a clue. Your friend says yes, and you both laugh again at the ridiculous episode—without boring her with an all too familiar tale.

My cousin told me that when she was over at a friend's for dinner the other night her hostess repeated the same story five times during the course of the evening. Aren't you glad you weren't there, and don't you hope it wasn't you?

One last thing about conversation: Don't forget to listen! I don't mean the "I can't wait until you finish to tell my side of it" kind. I mean *really* listen.

5. Humor

Lawrence Sterne said, in *The Case of Delicacy*, "I live in constant endeavor to fence against the infirmities of ill health and other evils of life by mirth, being firmly persuaded that every time a man smiles—but much more when he laughs, that it adds something to this Fragment of Life."

I firmly believe this. Below are what I believe to be the best types of humor to live by:

Laugh at yourself. The "I did the dumbest thing" kind of humor, if you can develop it, is, above all other forms, the most valuable.

Laugh at the tragicomic. When you spend the first two weeks in February in Florida, and it is 50 degrees every day, you can mope or you can laugh—you know which is better for you.

Everyone laughs at the ridiculous, but we each see the ridiculous in different things. I bought a new suitcase with small wheels hidden in the bottom and took it home on a bus. At the first sudden stop the suitcase rolled the whole length of the bus. As I laughingly chased it to the end I looked at the faces of the other passengers. Some were expressionless and others were laughing out loud. I couldn't help feeling sorry for those who could not find a minute to enjoy this ridiculous performance.

Exaggeration is my favorite kind: It can be a part of many kinds of humor, such as sarcastic, put-down, or whimsical, but it always gets a big laugh from me.

Whatever turns you on, laugh. You sometimes have a choice of laughing or crying. My neighbor dropped a gravy boat recently, splashing the brown, greasy contents all over my white rug, kitchen stove, refrigerator, and newly painted walls. While we were mopping and wiping she kept up these agonized groans. It got funnier and funnier until we both sat back on the floor convulsed in laughter. It was much more fun than crying. And, of course, all the stains came out anyway.

Laugh: It's much more fun and a lot better for you.

6. Toward Others

The "do unto others" teaching has been drummed into us so much that we don't hear it any more. Well, this ancient rule for living has been proven through the centuries, so let us take another look at it.

As we get older we either crawl deeper inside ourselves, losing our self-awareness, or open ourselves up through an interest in others. If you set out to help your friends you are the gainer, because you build up your pride. You gain more for yourself than you have given many times over. You don't even have to put yourself out very much.

The helping hand that involves volunteer work in hospitals, nursery schools, retirement homes is not so immediately rewarding. Extending yourself to a commitment of your time is a sacrifice you have to stop and think about. However, the move to help in a big way eventually pays off manyfold in enjoyment, pride, and a sense of accomplishment. On the worst icy day of the winter this year all the volunteers at a hospital showed up on time at 8:30 A.M. If these people could have developed such a commitment to their work that they drove through ice and snow when their only obligation was their own honor, doesn't this give you food for thought?

7. Characteristics to Take a Hard Look At

The personality problems you develop as you get older are really those that have always been there. They just become more intensified and rigid, unless self-awareness comes to your aid and helps you to control them. In this list of less favorable personality traits you may find one or two that will give you pause.

Self-pity. This is best overcome by activity. The term "wallowing in self-pity" is used with reason. Self-pity can so engulf you that there is no room for other thoughts. This is so self-destructive that your friends and relatives are in despair until you work out of it. Any interest outside of yourself will do, but you must get going.

Guilt. Remembering things in your life you think you should have done differently. Facing them is fine, but dwelling on them can only tear you down. Activity is again the answer. Get busy, so you have an interest to keep you from thinking about yourself all day.

Bossiness. Do you try to control everyone around you? Most devastating for children, others can avoid you.

Self-effacement. If you keep your annoyances inside, you build resentments. I know a man who spent a whole year hating the way his daughter-in-law cooked his eggs, a simple enough thing to change but he didn't want to hurt her feelings. When he finally suggested she flip his eggs, she flipped, and I mean literally. No harm done and this foolish problem, which had gotten out of all proportion in his mind, was easily solved.

Complaining. About your health, your lunch, your finances, or your neighbor are all boring to your listener if this is your constant attitude.

Blaming others for all of your problems. Get your self-awareness working to help you see this truth if you are guilty.

Perfectionism. This is such an ingrained characteristic that changing yourself probably won't work. The best thing you can do is to recognize that everyone is not going to share your need for perfection. Try humor on this one. If you are surrounded by a bunch of slobs, laugh.

Regression. This is a common development for some people as they get older. It is returning to the past, which is safe and known, rather than facing the present, which needs adjusting to. Keeping to the present by finding useful, pleasant things to do is a much happier choice.

Overindulgence. Women as well as men can try to drown their sorrows as their lives lose momentum and they begin to think of themselves as useless. If you fit into this picture, you had better see your doctor or Alcoholics Anonymous. There is nothing more disturbing to young people. I'll bet you have said, as many have, "I never want to be a burden to my children." This is a heavy burden.

8. Your Finances

I read a book recently, by Alan H. Olmstead, called *Threshold*. It is a fascinating diary started on the day before his retirement began and carried on through half a year. What threaded through the whole 192 days was a gnawing worry over money in a hard adjustment to living on less income.

Your financial situation, worrying as it is, can give you peace of mind or nagging worries in your retirement years. If you have an adequate income you are lucky. If you can see a struggle ahead, I vote for cutting back now. The authorities say you should slowly pull back in your living habits, so that the shock will be less when the income is lopped off. The saved money, of course, adds to the nest egg.

The saddest situation of all is to be confronted suddenly with financial decisions that you never have had to cope with before. "My husband always took care of everything." There is frustration, waste, and sometimes disaster in this situation. Now is the time to get yourself informed on taxes, wills, trust funds, the stock market, bonds. There are courses available, and your husband might even enroll, too.

A piece of advice I read recently was a suggestion on how to handle money in regard to your children, if you happen to have an excess. This financial authority warned against giving your adult children set sums of money on a regular basis (the government allows $3,000 per recipient per year without a gift tax). This man pointed out that they learn to expect it, don't appreciate it, and resent any cessation if you happen to want to use the money for something for yourself. Tax consultants may disagree. However, he advises to watch for a definite purpose and help out when it is needed. If Genevieve wants to go to Europe for the summer, you will be quite a heroine if you provide for the trip. Never turn all of your assets over to a member of the family to be doled out to you. You lose your self-esteem. Hold onto your purse strings as long as you are able.

If you expect a big cutback in living conditions, the next section provides some answers for retired happiness that don't cost a thing.

9. New Interests—Get Some!

A man in his early forties said to me the other day, "Since my father died, I have taken another look at my life and I am going to do everything now." How many things have we touched lightly upon, saying, "I'd like to learn this or do that someday." Someday is here. The more interests you can get to fill your time, provide you with new friends, and bolster your ego, the more fun you are going to have.

Here is a list of ten activities that will keep you busy.

a. *I always wanted to know what would happen if I put some paint on a canvas.* One day I passed an art supply store and I thought, "Why not?" I brought home sketchbook, charcoal, some brushes, and oil paints and started. This approach is not necessarily right. There are art schools that can give you proper instruction and make you a much better artist. I am lousy but enthusiastic. I knew a man once who had a heart attack, moved to Arizona, and became, from scratch, a well-know amateur in his community.

b. *Learn a musical instrument.* Playing a piano, violin, guitar can give you hours of pleasure. The challenge of learning is stimulating and the sense of accomplishment very satisfying. My mother's friend Margaret, who is in her late seventies, called one day and said, "Ann, I have lost my mind. I just bought myself a piano today. I used to play and I miss it." My mother's answer was, "Why not?" and it certainly was the right one.

c. *Change your decorating.* When was the last time you changed something in your home? If you have just let it sit there, think about it. It sparks the whole family to change the painted dining room walls to a patterned wallpaper. Learn to hang it yourself. Some comes prepasted, you know. If I can do it, you can. Take one room at a time and do a little something to it. My daughter moves the furniture every few months. It gives the old furniture a new look, and it certainly is inexpensive.

Within your budget you can dye the old bedspreads or buy new ones. You can have the dining room chairs recaned, or learn to do it yourself. Caning classes are available in most communities. Try painting the old chest of drawers and antiquing it. Antiquing glaze covers a multitude of sins. It may look so good you will want to buy new drawer pulls, available at most hardware and all big department stores.

Whatever you are inspired to do to spruce up the old place I guarantee will give you a big lift, and if you do it yourself the satisfaction is even greater.

d. *When I think of my beloved grandmother I always see her sewing.* She never sat down without her box of "pieces." She sewed little squares, diamonds, triangles of cloth together incessantly, for quilts, which her great-great-grandchildren are now sleeping under. Needlework is more durable than flesh and blood, so it is a satisfaction to know you are creating for posterity. Needlepoint has become the rage, but it can be very expensive if you buy the patterns. Try buying the backing and draw or trace your own pattern. I know someone who transferred a magazine cover of a very elaborate Victorian house. It is stunning. Another had an artist help her with duplicating the pattern in her Oriental rug for a three-paneled screen. Think of the fun you can have.

Knitting, crocheting, crewel, all can be a great satisfaction when finished and an interesting occupation in your spare time.

e. *There are stories in every high school and university of the grandmother who finished her degree at seventy.* I have one. When we were disposing of some of my mother's things, prior to a move, she called Clarabelle to offer her whatever she might want. Clarabelle had worked for my mother as a domestic but had retired several years before with a "misery" in her hip. As she was leaving with her loot my mother said, "Did you finish last year, Clarabelle?" Finish what? I found out. She had gone back to high school after she stopped working and in her late sixties had actually gotten her diploma.

High school or college level, there are courses to cover an infinite number of interests. From découpage to Dante you can find your niche. If you want to make your children proud of you, just take a course. "Do you know that my mother is studying differential calculus?" I have a friend, with two lawyer sons-in-law, who has just enrolled in a course called "para-law." Scares me to death to think of it when I can't even read an insurance policy.

f. *Church work.* When you are no longer needed at home on a twenty-four-hour basis, there is a great deal of satisfaction to be had from working in the women's group of the church of your choice. Contact with your fellowworkers provides new friends. Your esteem rises in yourself and is built up in your community. Joining in church activities is a great way to open doors if you relocate.

g. *Grow plants, or an herb garden.* If you have space, try organic vegetables. Maybe you love flowers. Exercise your green thumb, and talk to all of them lovingly.

The need to grow things is akin to having pets. The desire to care for something seems to show up strongest in the city of New York. The apartment population has gone berserk on plants and how decorative and how much fun they are!

h. *Hospitals are in constant need of volunteers.* They can be used from distributing the mail to preparing surgical dressings. Depending on the hospital, you can choose the kind of work you like best. Whether you work in the children's section of a hospital or in a nursing home it is a wonderful way to use your time.

i. *Lots of people enjoy following politics.* Strong emotions develop on issues and candidates. If this is your bag, don't just sit there. Volunteer. You may even end up marrying the candidate.

j. *Learn new games.* My mother, at eighty-seven played bridge three times a week and usually won. A contemporary of mine said,

"She was a better player than I am." Try bridge, canasta, backgammon, whatever can add a great deal to your life.

An older woman said to me one time, "The hardest thing about getting old is there is nothing to look forward to." I think your sights just get shorter. Certainly looking forward to being with friends for a game of bridge on Friday night can brighten up the whole week. Maybe you can't look forward to getting a medical degree but you can certainly learn a new game. I have just learned the new rage, the old game of backgammon. I wasn't an apt pupil and people still beat me constantly but it is sure fun.

Don't forget the outdoor games you were always going to learn and never got around to. They have the advantage of exercise and fresh air.

Golf is wonderful exercise and not strenuous. It is a great challenge to learn and most absorbing. There are golf pros to teach you at all public as well as private golf courses.

Tennis can be played at seventy. It is so terribly popular currently that you really will be in the swim with this one. Get a good instructor (professional) and learn the game well. You will have to develop consistency and accuracy, because you may not run as fast as your opponent.

Swimming is not a game but I am throwing it in here because the exercise is considered among the best. You really have to learn the strokes to get the most out of it, and that you can do at any YWCA or swim club.

10. Healthy Sex Attitudes

No matter what our age, we all like to be considered attractive to the opposite sex. Jean Baptiste Troisgros, a famous French restaurateur, is quoted as saying of women, when he was seventy-one, "At forty-five the devil takes over and they are beautiful, splendid, maternal, proud. The acidities are gone. When I see them my mouth waters."

One of my proudest moments occurred recently while I was hurriedly walking down a quiet side street in New York. Coming toward me was a bent old man, seemingly looking down at the sidewalk. As we came abreast he said, without lifting his head, "You sure got a beautiful pair of legs, woman." He shuffled on and I continued with an added lilt.

When a friend of mine found out I was writing a book for older women, her first comment was, "I hope you are going to include sex." I'll say I am. You can't have the complete story of any adult age group without including this drive that influences so many aspects of our lives.

Skipping other menopausal problems, let us consider its effect on your sex life. Physically, a woman in menopause and after should expect no change in her sexual interests. It is not uncommon, however, even in this day and age, for women to close off that part of their lives and put themselves on the old-age shelf. The psychologists say that the reason for this is the unconscious linking of the sex act with the ability to reproduce. When they no longer can bear children women think they no longer need sex. This attitude is disastrous. A vigorous sex life, for as long as possible, is necessary for both mental and physical health. The age of disinterest varies with the individual. Withholding sex at the menopause stage can wreck a marriage or send a heretofore faithful husband out scouting around.

With the present deluge of books on sexual subjects, it doesn't seem possible for any of us not to know a lot more than we were ever allowed to know before. The days of sex behind the bedroom door are over. Those of us who were never told about sex except by an older girl, who didn't know anything either, have taken this revolution with different attitudes. Some are in shock. But others are accepting young people's sexual freedom complacently. One couple I visited recently said in unison, "Look at all the fun we missed."

Regardless of your reaction, here are some pertinent facts that make sex from forty on a lot more understandable.

It has been clinically proven that the height of a woman's sexual drive is from thirty to forty. She declines at a very slow rate until she is in her sixties and can continue to be sexually active into her seventies. Taking the exercise and nutrition chapters in this book seriously can add sexual vigor at all ages. Individual differences can vary both ways. There can be two physical problems. One is a thinning of the vagina wall and the other is a loss of hormonal fluid. If a gynecologist is consulted, these problems can be helped with prescribed lubricants.

Physical problems are not always the main reason for inhibiting sex. The general attitude that sex is only for the young can affect the sexual life of older couples by causing guilt. The sexually alert in their seventies suppressed their interest in sexual relations because it was looked on as foolish. This "Go away, you old fool" thinking has been negated considerably by the present opening up of sex attitudes. Adult children of the widow or widower don't help much. They frown on actual dating and the thought of any hanky-panky is absolutely shocking, no matter what their own sexual behavior may be. The sexual revolution is not supposed to extend beyond forty—and never for an older relative.

Understanding the male problems in middle age can bring answers to puzzling behavior. The male sexual capacity starts to decline anywhere from eighteen to twenty, according to laboratory tests. By the time he is forty, there may be a noticeable incapacity, which frightens him. The male ego is so highly based on his sexual abilities that the first time he experiences an inadequacy he is devastated. Masters and Johnson, the generally accepted authorities on sex, say that only a small percentage of continuing impotency is caused by physical problems. The fear and anticipation of impotency is so great that this highly mind-controlled function is easily retarded. It need not be a problem if the couple talk about it and accept with humor the occasional failure. Easing the anxiety can make a continuing sex life possible.

It is not unusual for a male to hide his fear of impotency behind indifference. The female feels rejected and often suspects another woman. It is suggested that, after all the years of being chased, at this stage of the marriage the woman should become the aggressor. It has been proven that once a man has proof of his returned virility, he can usually carry on.

The study of the male climacteric has been neglected, because it is not a physical certainty like menopause. Some men have it and some men don't. Some have intense physical and emotional symptoms and some don't. The fact that it is so nebulous often leaves any unusual behavior of a male between forty and fifty-five undiagnosed.

Here are a few symptoms to look for if you are finding some unusual behavior in the male in your life: Quick to tire, no pep, irritability, memory lapses, and extreme nervousness. What to do? See a doctor. The cures are not perfected but studies are under way, which look good for the future. As for now, only a small percentage of men are affected.

The female emerging from menopause has greatly increased energy. She has a new zest for life, and it may be sexual. She can have the freedom from contraceptives, the Pill, the household teeming with children, which always placed sex behind the bedroom door and determined the time. This freedom can open up sex play that has been impossible before. A friend of mine confessed to me recently that she had never had sex in the daytime.

The extramarital fling is not new to the world. In grandpa's day it was just kept a lot quieter. Male infidelity, especially in the roving forties and fifties, when men need proof of their virility, is common knowledge. The woman of today, based on recent studies, is taking a few flings herself. Isolated examples always did. Women's Lib has liberated the younger modern woman in a lot of her thinking. The single standard we have been brought up on is slowly fading away. It is your own decision these days as to how you conduct your sex life.

If this chapter has started you thinking about yourself there is a lot more to come. Let's deal with your exterior self in the next chapter.

Bibliography

Bellak, Leopold. *The Best Years of Your Life*. New York: Atheneum, 1975.

Carnegie, Dorothy. *Don't Grow Old Grow Up*. New York: Dutton, 1972.

Donahue, Wilma and Tibbitts, Clark, eds. *Planning the Older Years*. Westport, Conn.: Greenwood Press, 1968.

Ginsberg, Norman and Kaufman, Irving, eds. *Normal Psychology of the Aging Process*. New York: International University Press, 1963.

Harris, Janet. *The Prime of Mrs. America*. New York: G. P. Putnam's Sons, 1975.

Jones, Doris and Jones, David. *Young until We Die*. New York: Coward, McCann & Geoghegan, 1973.

Olmstead, Alan. *Threshold*. New York: Harper & Row, 1975.

Sheldon, Alan, McEwan, Peter J. M., and Ryrser, Carol Pierson. *Retirement Patterns & Predictions*. DHEW Publication No. (ADM) 74–49, 1975.

Stoneycypher, D. D., Jr. *Getting Old & Staying Young*. New York: W. W. Norton, 1974.

2
Skin Care

"Beauty is in the eye of the beholder," as the old saying goes. What is the beholder looking for when he looks at you?

I have been confronted many times in my eighteen years as a model agent with a less-than-beautiful girl who thought she should be a model because her boyfriend thought she was pretty. Even the professionals in the photography business varied in their opinions. "Don't send me Janice, she's ugly," from one phone call and "I need Janice for this picture because she is the most beautiful girl in the city," from the next.

The Makua tribe thought their most beautiful woman was the one with the biggest lips, disfigured from childhood by hoops placed inside the mouth.

Our beholders are looking at our complexions. Even though your best chance of having nice skin is having a mother or grandmother with a gorgeous complexion, you can still be a beauty by bestowing tender loving care on what you've got. You can have a bad-looking skin at sixteen and improve it as you get older. Women at eighty can have a glowing complexion, wrinkles and all. Forget the wrinkles at any age and try for good color, good skin condition, and a pleasant expression. You can't look twenty again, but you can sure look a great fifty (sixty?).

Of the many millions of dollars spent in the United States each year on cosmetics, I'll bet some of it has come from your pocket. Let's take a look and see if it has always been spent in the right place.

Here is a rule of ten "do's" to give you a fine glowing complexion for the rest of your life:

1. Do you know your skin type. If it is dry, you certainly know it by now and have done things to correct it. Let's make sure you are doing the right things. Dry skin is the most common type, so you are among friends.

If your skin is normal, lucky you. Just make sure you preserve it carefully, because conditions can alter it. Too much wind and sun can dry and too much oil and fat in your diet can cause oily areas. Your skin is very much the reflection of your diet, so get to know the right foods for your skin type.

The combination of skin that is oily in the nose creases, forehead, and chin areas and dry in the cheeks and around the eyes is more complicated. Each area must be treated according to the condition. Keep the dry portions well protected with moisturizers and the oily areas well cleansed with fresheners.

2. Cleansing. Since we are concerned with keeping our skins young looking, let us consider our alternatives for a good rousing skin cleaning.

a. *Soap and water.* Use a good unscented soap, preferably a castile. You may want to go to a specialized skin soap, such as Neutrogena. Make a lather and apply with your fingertips in circular movements to the entire face and neck, all the way back beyond the ears. Rinse and rinse and rinse with warm water running from the tap. Rinse until the water is no longer slippery. Blot dry. Do this night and morning if your skin is relatively normal. If your skin is ultra dry or beyond middle age, you may want to skip the morning soaping and just rinse with warm water.

b. *Cleansing lotion.* Maybe you will find soap too drying and should shift over to a cleansing lotion. Look at the label to make sure it says "rinse off." If you remove it with tissue, some will remain on the skin. Buy a reputable name brand and keep away from fancy ingredients that won't take off any more dirt. If they claim to have moisturizer in them, don't let that sway you. It only washes off with the rinsing. Save that for later. If you are confused about what to buy, go to a large department store and ask for the representative of a cosmetic house you know. These women have been specially trained and should have the reputation of their line to uphold. If you take your chances on anyone who happens to be behind the counter, you may get someone from yard goods, sent down to fill in for the day. Believe me, I've had them.

Once you have found the right cleanser, use it at night and in the morning. If you are beyond middle age, as with soap, you may find your skin too sensitive for two washings. And, as with soap, just rinse with warm water. Don't ask me what middle age is. You'll have to let your skin, not your age in years, tell you that. I want to stress here the use of warm water. My first job at the age of seventeen was with a cosmetic firm. We were taught to use extremely hot water followed by ice wrapped in a towel "to close the pores." I later learned that pores can't be closed and violent contrasts can only be harmful to the skin.

c. *Baby oil, salad oil (yes!), or cleansing cream remove dirt and makeup if soaps and detergents prove too harsh for you.* Our problem here is to dissolve the film that remains after tissuing it off. The pores clog with the oil, retaining some of the dirt with it, unless followed by a freshener or an astringent. These tend to dry and moisturizer must be used immediately after.

3. Toning. Your face is clean. You have splashed it with water and now you need a freshener or an astringent. The freshener is primarily alcohol. The astringent has added chemicals and should not be used on a too delicate or aging skin. The fewer ingredients, including scents, in your freshener the better. You can even make your own with four parts of water to one part rubbing alcohol. To this I add one teaspoon of vinegar or lemon juice to adjust the acid mantle. This is a term bandied about by cosmeticians, which means that the ratio of alkaline and acid (PH factor) should be higher on the acid side for a good skin condition. Soaps and detergents are alkaline so, to restore the acid condition, a solution of vinegar or lemon juice, one teaspoon per cup of water, is a good idea. If you are using soap and not oils on your face, the water-vinegar (lemon juice) treatment may be a sufficient freshener for you.

4. Thinning. The skin is constantly replacing itself, sluffing off old, dry skin as new cells are formed. To insure the complete removal of all of the dead skin and avoid a blotchy complexion it is necessary to use some mechanical, chemical, or abrasive treatment. The simplest is a terry washcloth used with vigor over the face and neck. This is good for the very young and those with troubled skin. The older skin may, however, need stronger methods. There are chemical thinners that are usually peels. When they are allowed to dry, they are washed off, taking the old skin with them. These work very well for the purpose but are inclined to dry the skin. Abrasive creams are very effective. They contain small particles of pumice or ground almonds and sometimes oatmeal and are also left on the skin until dry and then washed off, taking the dead skin with them. The loofa is a most effective mechanical method for thinning, and it is harmless for older skin. It would seem to rub the skin right off your face but, with relatively normal skin, it feels smooth as silk afterwards. Your skin becomes thicker as you get older, so it can tolerate this vigorous treatment. Watch under the eyes, however, as the skin there is of a different texture. If the whole procedure seems too strenuous for your skin, use the other methods.

The loofa cloth is a natural fiber that comes in a long, cigar-shaped piece, a flat, terry-backed pad, and recently has appeared in two kinds of mitts. One consists of natural fiber on one side and terrycloth on the other. The other is a knitted mitt with a combination of loofa fibers and cotton cord.

How often should you thin your face? Dr. Bedford Shelmire, Jr., in his book *The Art of Looking Younger,* recommends twice a week from middle age on. If you are younger, you can thin three times a week to advantage.

Warning: Do not expose your skin to the sun, wind, or severe cold directly after thinning. You have removed a layer of skin. Dead or not, it protects against the elements. You must wait until the natural oils have been replenished.

5. Moisturizing. Use a moisturizer immediately after whichever of these cleansing, freshening, or thinning routines you have chosen. If your skin is excessively dry, splash a little more water on your face after the freshener and pat it dry. The older you are the better it is to use a heavier moisturizer. You should use yours directly after your morning cleansing, before your makeup. Use one that will disappear into the skin, leaving no oily surface, but heavy enough to give a resiliency to the touch. I thought I needed a heavier consistency recently, so I tried a well-known brand-new product. Disaster! I was an oily mess. The next purchase disappeared into my skin leaving no resiliency at all. Until finally, like Goldilocks, I found one that was "just right." If you think I abandon all the wrong, costly products I buy, you are wrong. I combine them. Try this with color cosmetics too. Too pink? Add some of that too-orange you bought last month and you may have it.

Be sure to use a heavier moisturizer at night. Creams with all those exotic and intriguing names are unnecessary. Something dense and coating, which will hold in the moisture, will do the trick. I use vaseline at room temperature and wipe off the excess to save the bed linens and my hair. Your face feels wonderful in the morning. Be sure to remove it thoroughly before applying your makeup.

The action of all creams and oils is to lubricate and soften the skin. They also provide a film that keeps the natural moisture within the skin. That is all we can expect from creams and lotions. There are no miracle wrinkle removers that have any permanent effect.

The skin is made up of three layers: a) the epidermis, b) the dermis, and c) the subcutaneous layer. The epidermis is the outer layer visible to all and can be cleansed, softened, and protected by you. The dermis contains the blood vessels that carry the blood to the outer skin—and let it be of good quality, based on good nutrition, for a glowing skin. It contains connective tissue. Here is a problem area as your skin gets older. Elasticity, due to cross-linkage of collegen, the connective substance, decreases with the years. This is speeded up by deterioration from the sun, pollution, and thoughtless damage done in earlier years. The dermis also contains nerves, hair follicles, and oil glands. It is pretty obvious with all that going on just under your visible, thin skin that it better be protected from the above deteriorations at all times.

The lower level is the subcutaneous layer, where your serious problems really come from. This firming, supporting layer disintegrates as you get older, forming the deeper lines you would like to do without. Feeding our cells with good nutrients is the best way to slow down this deterioration. What you put on top isn't going to do it. Creams and lotions cannot penetrate to this level.

6. Exercise your face. This is highly contested by dermatologists, and I must agree that I cannot see how the muscles can lift the sagging outer layers of the skin. I do think, however, that you can control your expression to make you a more pleasant-appearing person. The scalp and forehead muscles can be exercised to control frown lines. The facial muscles, both horizontal and vertical, can keep those droopy mouth corners up. If you develop an awareness of the muscles that control these important expression areas, you are on the road to improvement. If either one is allowed to become your permanent look, you can appear constantly worried with frowning, or unhappy, disillusioned, or downright mean with your mouth sagging at the corners. Look around at some of your friends.

EXERCISES FOR THE FROWN:

a. Pull the muscles back right at the hairline. Hold for five counts and relax. Repeat five times twice a day. You can do this any time or place, since it is scarcely noticeable.

b. Lift your eyebrows up as high as they will go, being aware of a sideward pull. These are two separate muscles. First up and then out. Hold ten counts. Repeat five times.

You can exercise your face forever and not accomplish anything unless you apply these exercises in everyday living, which is the point. Right? When someone spills chocolate ice cream on your new white rug, don't frown. Pull the muscles at the hairline. Lost your keys? Don't frown, try the other pocket.

The lower part of the face is the first to age. Gravity pulls those corners down, down, down. The cheeks fall, forming a groove from nose to mouth. Mouth corners to chin collapse in a groove of flesh, which causes those unpleasant expressions you don't want.*

EXERCISES FOR THE CHEEK MUSCLES:

a. Teeth clenched, lips together; now pull the muscles up, up, up at the corners. You will be using two sets of muscles, those in the cheeks and those at the sides of the mouth. Hold ten counts and repeat five times. This can be done on alternate sides of the face by opening the lips at one corner and pulling up, then the other corner, holding ten counts on each side, five times a side.
b. Lips together, teeth apart, place the tip of your tongue against the inside of your lower teeth. Push with the tongue raising the upper lip muscles and cheek muscles. I do this ten times a day, or whenever I think of it. Pull up those corners!

Just for good measure, and just in case it can do some good, let me tell you about an eye exercise that some people swear by. Look into the mirror for this one. Squint your eyes, pulling the lower lid up as hard as you can. See the sag under the eyes disappear? The

---

*If you are forty, there may be little telltale grooves starting. If you are sixty, they are probably well established.

theory is that if you start young enough you can forestall these circles, and if you start at any time you can't cure them but you can slow down the additional future sagging.

7. Remove blemishes. If you have moles or any other kind of growth on your face, you are not the one who has to look at them. Ask your doctor about how to proceed. How the removal will be handled depends on the kind of growth, of course. It can be done surgically, chemically, or electrically. I recently had a very small cyst removed by a plastic surgeon in his office in ten minutes and walked out without a bandage on my nose. Certainly no scar. Of course, you know you should see your doctor, if there is any color, texture change, or enlargement of any existing growth, for cancerous possibilities. Other growths to watch for are yellow plaques on the eyelids. These are unsightly and easily removed. Small warts are not uncommon. If they are in a prominent place, do something about them.

The flat brown spots, which we always call "liver spots," aren't caused by any liver disorder at all. These are more difficult to deal with surgically but sometimes they respond to bleach creams. One that is one of the oldest on the market and has given me good results is Esoterica. The ones to avoid contain mercury. Look on the label before buying one. In any event, do not apply to a large area before trying a patch test to see if your skin can tolerate it. The younger you are the more effective the cream, so start early with the first sign.

8. Remove or bleach unsightly excess hair. Due to the hormone imbalance after menopause, facial hair can become excessive on the upper cheek, the upper lip, or the chin. The only permanent removal is by electrolysis. It is safe and completely destroys the hair follicle. The oldest school for training operators is the Kree Institute in New York City. They have been working with electrolysis for fifty-five years and have trained operators from all over the world. The problem with electrolysis is that there is no safe way to estimate the time and cost of eliminating the hair. Niles Dorian, the director of the institute, points out the problem: "Neither patient nor operator can estimate how many hairs are in a given area." Please watch any advertising that guarantees removal of all hair on your upper lip in a given period. The average cost for most operators is twenty-five dollars an hour and the average treatment is fifteen minutes. Never, never try any do-it-yourself kits. You just can't control the equipment on yourself.

Waxing is a process in which a special wax is heated and applied by a competent operator. It is allowed to harden and then peeled off, taking the hairs with it. It will be effective from four to five weeks. It is used sometimes on excessively dense eyebrows also.

Depilatories are dependable for removing excess hair from any part of the body. They are drying and must be followed by a good moisturizer. They do not impede the growth of hair but remove the hair closer than shaving. Never shave the face or arms. If there is hair on arms, legs, or thighs, which is unsightly but should not be shaved, the use of a peroxide solution should be considered. It will lighten the color, making the hair less noticeable. Try a solution of four parts water to one part peroxide and reduce the water if you don't get adequate results in the first try. When you apply it, make sure it stays on top of the hairs and does not lie on the skin underneath.

Watch the hair in your nostrils. These tend to grow more actively as you get older. Depending on the construction, the nostril exposure is greater in some people than others. Visible hairs in the open nostrils are not pretty and can be removed by tweezing or electrolysis.

9. Do know about dermabrasion. This is a process that removes the surface skin, which eliminates brown spots and surface lines. If you are in the public eye and need to keep your looks up to snuff, this may be a helpful process for you. It requires a hospital visit of two to three days, along with a red face for two to three weeks. A good plastic surgeon, recommended by your doctor, is the only one to trust with this treatment. A closely related method called chemo-surgery is a strong chemical applied to the skin; this should also be done by a plastic surgeon. Mostly, it is done only in certain areas of the face in comparison with dermabrasion, which is a full face treatment.

Silicone injections to fill in the skin under the wrinkles is not to be considered as it is prohibited by the Food and Drug Administration, and for good reason. The silicone can move from the original point of injection and lodge in areas where you don't need or want plumping up, such as under the eyelids. Worse than that, it can move to more vital organs and cause even more serious trouble.

10. Face-lifting. This is an entirely personal decision and should be considered carefully. Pick a well-known, reputable plastic surgeon in your community. If you are in doubt, call a good hospital and ask for a list of plastic surgeons on their staff. Make an appointment for an interview. A good doctor will not rush into anything. He will want to know how your husband feels about it, how much you expect from it. It seems to be quite a common problem that many patients expect to turn into Liz Taylors, even though they were Zasu Pitts types to begin with. It is definitely surgery, with at least five days in the hospital and two to three weeks out of circulation. The average length of effectiveness is five years. The cost is high, depending on your locality, and can vary from doctor to doctor.

Here are ten "don'ts" for better skin:

1. The biggest "don't" of all is sun exposure. Dermatologists scream their loudest about the aging effects of too much sun. The sebaceous glands in the dermis layer of the skin provide the oil that forms a protective coating for the epidermis. When subjected to too much sun, these glands are not able to provide enough oil to counteract the drying effects of the sun and the damage is to all three layers of the skin.

As the skin ages, another problem develops. The skin is developing the liver spots we spoke of before. When subjected to the sun, these spots darken and develop even more. The sun also causes rough red spots on some people, which should be removed since they are not only ugly but precancerous.

Red spots, liver spots, or not, I love the sun. None of us want to stay home under the bed when everyone else is out in the strong sun rays ruining their skin and having fun. What to do! Luckily cosmeticians have been working with this problem for quite awhile and have produced a number of sun screens that are very helpful. Look for one that contains paraminobenzoic acid. Redheads can go into the sun for the first time in their lives with this screen copiously coating them. The only problem with it is that it stains. I found this out the hard way by ruining my favorite beach robe. It didn't rub off of my skin but leaked out of the bottle. Watch your white bathing suits or tennis dresses. Other effective ingredients to look for on the label are benzobonone derivatives or salicylates. Slather the stuff on. If you swim or perspire, slather it on repeatedly. Wear a hat! Cover yourself in the middle hours of the day with a towel or long-sleeved shirt. Don't sunburn! Blisters can leave unsightly scars for months.

If you are a skier you are in triple trouble. You not only have the sun reflecting from the snow, there are also the wind and the extreme cold, all are drying factors. Carry your bottle with you and apply copiously all day. The friend who stands out in my mind as having the most prematurely aged skin is a skier. Be it boating, tennis, the beach, or skiing, run right back to your quarters and use the heaviest moisturizer you can get.

Repeat from "do" number 4. Don't go into the sun, wind, or cold directly after using a mask or thinner on your skin.

2. Don't live in a heated house or apartment without some kind of humidifier. Enough trouble can develop to make the purchase of a furnace or room humidifier worthwhile. If you already have one on your furnace, you may want to put a small unit in another room in the house. I like mine in the room where I sleep. After all, I am there eight hours—most nights. Our skin needs all the moisture it can get to keep it soft and glowing. Give it all you can.

There are several sizes of room humidifiers, depending on the number of gallons they hold. It's up to you how many times you want to fill it and how much you can afford to pay for it. I have a friend who complains all winter long about her itchy, dry skin and refuses to consider a $10.00 purchase, which would eliminate the trouble. Units range in price from $10.00 to $60.00, according to model, store, and community.

3. Don't forget the skin on the rest of your body. That ages right along with your face and is just as telltale. You use a hand lotion frequently, I'll bet. What about your arms? What about your legs? They are exposed to the drying conditions of the elements and heated rooms, too. Be sure to use a good lotion or cream with a lanolin base to keep that moisture in on all your visible surfaces.

4. Don't rely on masks for any wrinkle curing that is permanent. Masks act as an additional moisturizer, sealing in the moisture. They are made up of clay, synthetic rubber, and other materials that harden, causing the skin to swell slightly. After removal, the skin is plumped up for a short time, and it's fun. Someone said one time, "I have yet to see a woman walk out of a beauty parlor who didn't look as if she believed it." But it is of short duration.

5. Don't feed your skin, feed yourself. The skin is fed by the bloodstream and must get the right nutrients from it to maintain good texture and color. If your eating habits are bad, you probably don't realize that the results are showing up in your complexion. You may be treating it fine from the outside, with all kinds of creams and lotions, but the actual color or glow is missing. Remember that your face pales when you are sick? What goes on inside shows on the outside.

Here are some of the vitamins that affect the skin:

> B-2 and PABA (para-ambinzenoic acid) for discoloration and blotches. Small amounts of PABA are included in most B complex tablets. See your doctor for any larger amounts, as you needed a prescription.
> A for softer, smoother skin.
> C, A, F (linoleic and lanolenic acids) for dry skin.
> C, lecithin, for elasticity and resistance to infections.
> E, B complex, lecithin, F, for resistance to wrinkles.

Until you get the whole story in chapter 5, eat plenty of protein, drink your orange juice, and eat plenty of leafy vegetables. Eat whole-grain breads and make sure you get plenty of iron.

6. Don't lose weight too fast. Take away the supporting fat cells and your skin will sag. The elasticity of your skin diminishes as you get older and it cannot keep its contour as readily. With a slower loss of weight, based on good nutrition, the skin can adjust.

7. Don't ignore a sudden skin problem. Think of any new cosmetic you may be using. Maybe you are taking a new medication. Many drugs react badly on the skin. Don't forget possible irritation from fabrics: wool, dyes, and tight-fitting garments that rub against the skin can cause trouble. It took me three years to throw a dress out. It never dawned on me that every time I wore that green wool dress I began to itch all up and down my arms. One day a dark red blotch appeared and I began to see the light. Out it went and my problem with it. I never will know whether it was that particular wool or that particular dye.

8. Don't ignore the small blood vessels that may be surfacing. Anything that causes the viewer to look at a less-than-beautiful you should be attended to. If you have slight surfacing in one or two areas, these can be covered with a heavier foundation of the same tone but a shade darker than your regular base. Cover the area before and after using the lighter base. If you are really afflicted with dark and numerous surface vessels, see your doctor. He can recommend a dermatologist who can remove them with a fine electric needle. Insist on a dermatologist.

9. Don't listen to Mabel, who has just found the most wonderful new product, which may not be for you at all. As I said, know your skin type and don't get carried away in the wrong direction. It can save you a lot of money.

10. Don't buy skin care items for their fancy ingredients. The simplest and purest are the best and serve the same purpose. You can even make your own. Virginia Castleton Thomas has written a book giving skin care recipes going back through the centuries. It is called *My Secrets of Natural Beauty*. The age-old recipes for masks, bleaches, cleansers, and moisturizers are from such simple household items as vinegar, honey, egg white, buttermilk, heavy cream, lemon, and on and on. New York models have taken to using yogurt as a facial mask, and it is worth a try. It makes your face feel wonderful after it has been rinsed off with warm water. (No strawberry or apricot, please, just plain yogurt.)

Remember that your face is what the beholder sees first and deserves all the care you can give it.

> If to her share some female errors fall,
> Look to her face, and you'll forget 'em all.
> —"The Rape of the Lock"
> Alexander Pope

Don't you wish!

Bibliography

Archer, Leslie. *Let's Face It*. Philadelphia: J. B. Lippincott Co., 1965.

Baker, Aleda. *Models' Way to Beauty, Slenderness and Glowing Health*. Englewood Cliffs, N.J.: Prentice-Hall, 1973.

Crenshaw, Mary Ann. *The Natural Way to Super Beauty*. New York: McKay, 1972.

Ford, Eileen. *Secrets of the Models' World*. New York: Simon & Schuster, 1970.

Hauser, Gaylord. *Mirror, Mirror, on The Wall*. New York: Fawcett, Crest, 1961.

———. *The Art of Being Beautiful at Any Age*. New York: St. Martin's Press, 1975.

Shelmire, J. Bedford. *The Art of Looking Younger*. New York: St. Martin's Press, 1973.

Sternberg, Thomas. *More Than Skin Deep*. New York: Doubleday, 1970.

Thomas, Virginia Castleton. *My Secrets of Natural Beauty*. New Canaan, Conn.: Keats, 1972.

3
Makeup, False Eyelashes and All

Charles Kettering said, "If you have always done it that way, it is probably wrong."

Maybe you haven't changed your makeup since you dabbed on that first lipstick against your mother's violent protests. Since those days makeup has entered the fashion world. Changes come with fashion trends. First it's the thin eyebrow and then its the natural and back again. Bright red lipstick was replaced by very soft colors, very soft. (A girl in my office during this vogue used three light shades on top of one other and then covered them all with white.) The eyebrows and lips are the two most obvious areas, but there are more. You change your skirt length, why not your makeup? Beyond a certain age, to follow the exaggerated look of a high-fashion model is bizarre. But a modified nod to the current fashion is going to be noticed and admired by your younger friends and colleagues.

The use of makeup is a relative thing. Where do you live? Is your community wearing eyeliners this season? What is your social life and structure? What is your personality? A dramatic, highly fashionable woman I knew wore considerable makeup into her late seventies. That was Lillian and she looked great. I think that most women can improve their appearance with more makeup, skillfully applied, and in the right colors. The trap here is when to quit. I found that most new models who were experimenting with makeup would get heavier and heavier handed until I would have to bring them back to normal after a few months.

The cosmetic world has fascinated me since my first job at a makeup counter at the age of eighteen. My business as a model agent for eighteen years was very much involved with makeup. Many beautiful and many pretty plain faces had to have help. I learned a lot of tricks to bring out the best features in all shapes and complexions.

Here are ten "do's" for better makeup, which I hope will help you on the road to becoming a more beautiful mature woman:

1. Do make up in the proper light. A friend of mine said to me the other day, "I hate you. Ever since you told me to make up at the window I see all the wrinkles." Never mind the wrinkles you see. It's more important to see what others are seeing. Use daylight directly on your face. You are not applying eye shadow for a cozy tête-à-tête in a dark restaurant every time you leave the house. You can probably benefit from a magnifying mirror. They come in purse size, table stands, and one beauty that stands on the floor and adjusts to face level. The wall-mounted type that swings out works fine, but it may be hard to find a good place to hang it. There are special magnifying, extended glasses and some now that fit over your own glasses, which allows for using your regular mirrors. Just make sure you see your face in detail and have both hands free.

Every time I say this I picture a girl I saw on a bus one day. She brought a bottle out of her purse and calmly covered her face with foundation; next a jar from which she deftly applied her eye shadow. Rouge, lipstick, and mascara followed—all without ever looking in a mirror. She popped off the bus hopefully on time for her appointment. An actress? Certainly someone who knew makeup. Let's not try that.

After you have your makeup on, check it with a regular mirror in artificial light. You can sometimes see that the overall effect is not what you want. Make your corrections in this light.

2. Your face is clean and you have applied moisturizer. Now comes the important color foundation. It is sometimes called the base. Always use the moisturizer first, as the pigment in the foundation can clog the pores and even show up as individual dots if the pores are enlarged.

"Why do I need a base?" I would be asked quite often by some young beauty who had not used much makeup before. It has the necessary advantage of giving the face a uniform color. You may be showing some discoloration in certain areas, small brownish spots, or larger "liver spots." Foundation can tone them down. It is also easier to apply your other makeup over a base. Rouge, eye shadow, corrective makeup smooth on easier. Lips lose their firm line as you get older and small lines sometimes appear around the mouth. If the foundation is brought over the edges of the lips, the mouth line can be defined better and the lipstick will not bleed into the lines. A foundation is also an additional protection against sun, wind, cold, dirt, and pollution.

The two important things to look for in choosing a foundation are color and density:

COLOR:

a. Check the color you have been wearing and make sure it is the same as your own skin tone.
b. Don't accept any color a salesgirl suggests. Try it first on your neck and not the back of your hand. The skin on the hand is not the same texture or color as your face. Try to get to daylight to see the color. Check to make sure that you can return it if it is all wrong.

c. Keep away from too dark or muddy a color. This goes for black skin too. Keep the tones soft.
d. Keep away from too pink or too orange. I don't know why some people wear these shades.
e. Change your color when your tan goes. A phony tan can look mighty peculiar with a white neck.
f. Too light a color can give a pasty look on the wrong skin. I had a model once who got all kinds of complaints from the customers for using too much makeup. We worked toning everything down and still had the problem. Finally I had her try a little more color in her foundation and the problem was solved. Your makeup will appear stronger, too, on a white skin. I ought to explain here that this is the only cheating to another shade than your own skin tone that is good, and then it has to be chosen with extreme care. I even believe that there is nothing wrong in upping the color after an illness, when you are definitely pale. Here you can look mawkish if you go overboard, though.
g. Maybe you have experimented with a colored toner used under the foundation. Most makeup lines carry them and they are effective on some skins. They come in a green for the too-florid complexion and mauve for the sallow. These are best used in such areas of the face as under the eyes or cheeks. I have seen pretty artificial effects from all-over application.

TEXTURE:

A thinner base should be used as lines start to appear, contrary to the "let's cover them up" impulse. The denser base lays in the lines, making them appear deeper. You might want to try a colored moisturizer, which gives a soft glow and appears like no makeup at all. Pick this one very carefully. This is not for everyone, as it is extremely light textured. Change your foundation once in awhile. You may feel you have the perfect color and texture for yourself and wouldn't change it for the world. How do you know? Maybe there is something new on the market that is that much better. Maybe your skin has changed slightly since you started using this one. A new makeup item is a great morale booster.

3. Now is the time to think of covering any lines. Have on hand a lighter-colored base, a little bit heavier in texture. It can be at least three shades lighter. I do not mean one of those "hide it" sticks. Heaven forbid. They give a caked look to even very young skins. Apply this lotion (it should be a lotion) to such wrinkled areas as those beneath the eyes, the crow's feet, and the line from the nose to the chin, where the sagging mouth line develops. Apply it before the foundation and after. Blend it carefully so that it blends in and doesn't look like a light streak. Never use white, it is too strong. This lighter base can be used several times a day and before going out at night, if there is no time for a complete new makeup. Be sure that you are not getting a caked-looking buildup.

4. Eyebrows are your most important facial feature, next to your eyes because they can control your expressions. I have changed a lot of eyebrow lines in my years of working with models. Here are some of the things I found to be important:

a. Pluck the hairs underneath the brow and where they straggle out at the end. Those hairs that do not form some kind of line give you an untidy appearance.
b. Consider the shape of your eyes and the position of your brow bone before you start to shape your eyebrows. Proceed with caution, taking only a couple at a time, because the tiniest change can make all the difference.
c. Here are some of the common structural problems to consider when you are forming your eyebrows:
 1) Brow bone too close to the eye. Remove the hairs beneath the eyebrow to open up the eye. This problem is usually better solved with an arch. Experiment.
 2) High brow bone, which can cause a slightly startled expression. Pluck from the top and follow the bone line if it isn't too arched. A straighter brow is better here.

Common Structural Faults

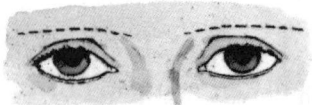 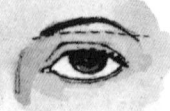

LOW BROW
Pluck hairs beneath brow and
add color at top to form
slight arch

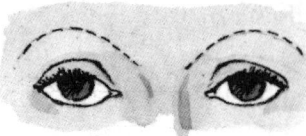 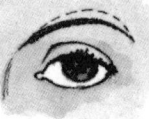

HIGH BROW
Pluck top hairs of brow and
pencil in lower edge to form
a straighter line

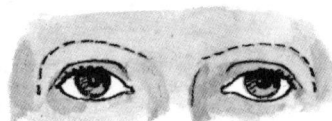 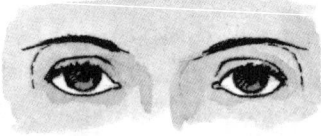

BROW CLOSES IN AT SIDES
Pluck hairs that grow down, closing
in the eyes, and pencil in a
horizontal line

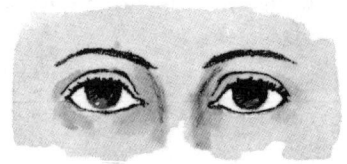 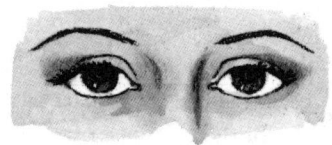

EYES TOO CLOSE TOGETHER
Pluck hairs near nose bridge, extending brow
color outward from the corner of the eye

3) The nicely arched brow bone that drops abruptly, closing in the eye at the outer edge. Pluck the hairs at the end so that they do not follow the bone.
4) Eyes too close together. Pluck your eyebrows out from the nose bridge. Hold a pencil perpendicular to the corner of your eye, and cheat out from that line. (By the way, with eyes normally spaced, this is where the eyebrow should begin, directly above the corner.)
5) Eyes too far apart. This is usually not a problem, as the eyes give a nice expression with this structure. Occasionally the proportions are out of balance and then the brows should be shortened at the outer edge and brought closer to the bridge of the nose.

d. Keeping in mind that eyebrows are important for a pleasant expression, you will now probably find it necessary to add to them. If they are short after the plucking, draw them out. Too close to the eyes? Draw a slight addition to the top line. You can form an arch. You can straighten them. Just keep them right for your looks.

e. There are pencils and powders to work with. I like a soft brown cake powder, which I apply with a short-handled brush. The sable bristles have been slanted for forming a narrower line. They cost around $2.50, are washable, and will last forever. If you use a pencil, apply it with short strokes, as though you were drawing hair. See that the pencil does not leave a shiny effect.

f. Keep the color you add soft and close to the hair on your brunette head. Blonds or redheads with light eyebrows will want to darken them with soft brown or mushroom. Black hair sometimes is fine with black brows, but age and skin tone will sometimes call for softening to a lighter brown.

g. If your eyebrows are terribly black and bushy, and you have a daily problem of keeping them neat, you may want to resort to electrolysis. A competent operator can advise you. You can have the strong black toned down by dyeing, done in a beauty salon by a good technician. This is for newly made blonds or redheads. If your hair is grey or white and the brows are still black you can soften your expression with a lighter color. Peroxide works for some people. Try a weak solution and graduate to a stronger one until you get results. Keep the solution on your brows, not the skin, and don't let it run into your eyes.

h. Your eyebrows may be all nicely plucked into a lovely arch and you may still have the problem of some curly, bristly hair that just won't stay put. Most cosmetic companies put out an eyebrow fixative for these nonconformers.

i. My pet peeves:
  Eyebrows that start with a heavy blunt line.
  Eyebrows that curve way down at the outer edge.
  Eyebrows that arch in a fine line halfway up the forehead.
  A sharp, fine line that is drawn where an eyebrow should be.
  Eyebrows that are very bushy over the nose bridge.
Look around you. You will see them all.

5. Eyeshadow comes in powdered form, cake, or creams. It comes in an unending variety of colors. From this distance, I can only help you with a few suggestions. We are involved with your eye shape, brow bone, eye set, and skin tone. So where do we start?

Taking them in order: your choice between powder and cream is your own. If you like cream, be sure to get one that isn't greasy. A shiny lid is unnatural. Explore a greaseless cream that is now on the market, so the color won't lie darkly in the creases. The powder or cake is never shiny and stays on better for me. Your color choices are just as good in one as the other.

COLOR:

The safest color for an older eyes is a soft light brown or mushroom. This is the color of the eyelid skin, slightly exaggerated. If, however, you are used to color, you can tone it down with a little brushed-on brown or beige powder. The point of eyeshadow is to enhance the eye itself and not draw attention to the eyelid with

My Pet Eyebrow Peeves

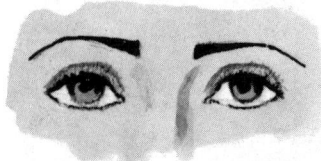

Eyebrows that start with a heavy blunt line

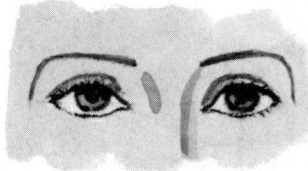

Eyebrows drawn down at the outer edge

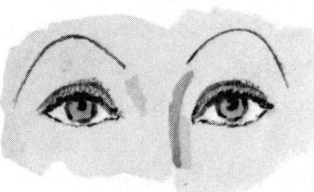

Eyebrows arched in a fine line halfway up the forehead

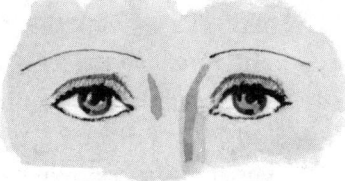

Entire brow plucked and artificial fine line drawn

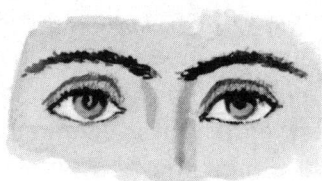

Bushy eyebrows growing onto the bridge of the nose

bright blues and greens. The use of beige for the crinkled eyelid softens the crinkles. There is also a pink shadow used at present, which might be right for you if your complexion is on the rosy tones.

EYE SHAPES:

- a. Round. The round eye can be attractive, open, and friendly, but sometimes it needs to be flattened down a little if the expression is starey. Keep the shadow heaviest at the center of the lid directly above the pupil.
- b. Slitting eyes. Keep the dark line well back on the lid and carry it back to the crease. Use a light color nearest the eye.
- c. Small eyes. Keep the dark color back to the crease and the lighter next to the eye but carry them both out beyond the eye. Be careful to blend the two so there will be no sharp line where they meet.
- d. Eyes that drop down at the ends. Concentrate the lighter color from the center of the eye beyond the outside and the darker back to the crease and to the corners.
- e. Deep-set eyes. Lighten the back of the lid to the crease and carry it up to the brow bone.
- f. The flat eye. The eye that doesn't sit back into a noticeable socket can be dropped back with a dark shadow covering the whole lid. A stronger dark line can be run along where a crease normally is. Use a lighter line directly under the eyebrow. The use of dark next to light in all makeup augments the effects of both. Where the two meet they must be carefully blended.

There are many variations of these basic shapes, so that you may not find yourself in any one of them. Knowing the principle of light standing out and dark dropping back you can work out your problem for yourself.

6. Eyeliner is subject to fashion changes. Several years ago shiny liquid liners were in. They produced a strong line, which did not always produce a pleasant expression, however. The pendulum has swung to almost no liner and heavy mascara. This is quite nice and is used to help the shape of the eye with a soft, blended line above

Eye Shapes

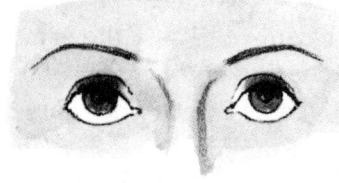

Round

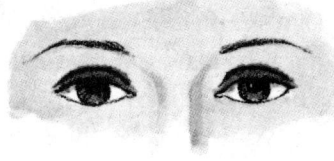

Slitting

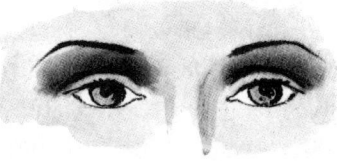

Small

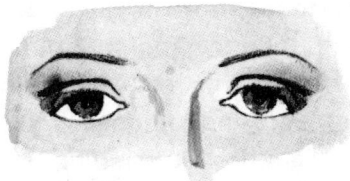

Angling downward

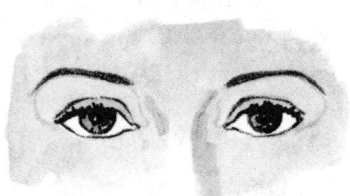

Deep-set

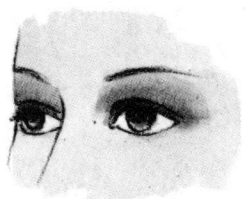

Flat

and on the lower lid. This can be in color and if carefully chosen and cleverly applied will bring out your own eye color.

Here let's pause to take a look. If you have been using the same liner for years, maybe it is too strong for your face and hardens your expression. These new soft powders, applied with a fine-tipped brush, are very good for the forty and older group.

7. Mascara. Black, brown, or blue are the only colors we should consider. I am very nervous about mascara because I always see it instead of the eyes when used too heavily. I especially notice it with those who are wearing glasses when the magnified mascara is more obvious. I feel that mascara during the day must be used with discretion. If you work all day in artificial light in a fashion-oriented occupation, you will probably want to wear some. Everyone else does. But on the golf course, the tennis court, or beach, it is bound to be more apparent. If you do use it during the day, blot it with your thumb and forefinger while it is still wet, to separate the lashes.

At night, in your shining best, it can be very alluring. You may want to use two coats but avoid beading by blotting again with your fingers.

8. False eyelashes. Buy a very sparse strip, cut a smidgen shorter than your eyelid. Don't let everyone know they are false by wearing too heavy or too coarse an eyelash. Get surgical adhesive from any drugstore or cosmetic counter. Apply it to the strip and press on as close to your own lashes as possible. If you ever use a liner, use one now. Use it before you put on the lashes and apply a little wider than you ordinarily would. This softens the strip line and fills in if you don't get the lashes as close to your own as you should. It is lots of fun and you feel like Marlene Dietrich. Don't forget to mascara as the final touch to work the two, old and new, together.

There is a salon in New York, run by Jean Kane, who does a big business in applying lashes individually. It takes about an hour, costs about $25.00, and they stay on about two weeks. They say there is a Prince Charming around the corner waiting for you at any age. Maybe for that special occasion you are going to? Who knows?

9. Rouge. Here again we have liquid powders and creams to choose from, and color galore. Between powders and creams, I take creams. They don't blotch on any irregularity on the skin or cake on foundation that hasn't absorbed. They come in stick form (blushers), pots, and pressed neatly into compacts. They do have a tendency to fade and may need to be reapplied during the day.

COLOR:

Keep away from all purplish, bluish tones. With that warning, I can't help you much further. Your own skin tone dictates the color and your skin chemistry controls how it ends up after it gets on the skin. Earth tones are fashionable and by that I mean they have a lot of brown in them. They go on very naturally, but avoid the too-dark shades.

Where? For years I never wore rouge. I abhored those pink dots on every cheek. Recently I have been talked into wearing one of the soft earth shades and I see the improvement. Rouge these days is being worn higher and away from the nose, depending on the shape of your face.

Pick your face shape:

a. If your face is long, keep the rouge just below the cheek bone and bring it onto the cheek, breaking up the length half way.
b. If your face is round, keep the rouge closer to the center of the cheek in an oval pattern.
c. The square face. Start the rouge at the cheekbone and cheat the line to a definite inward slant. Round it half way into the cheek, forming a curve back to the bone in front of the ear. Taper off the color as you go back.
d. The oval face; the prized one. From above the cheek bone form a triangle. How far you come down on your face with the point depends on the length of your face.

Rouge
(Pick Your Own Face Shape)

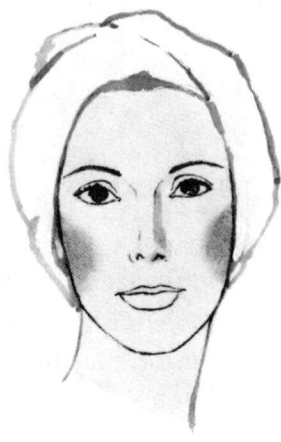

Oblong

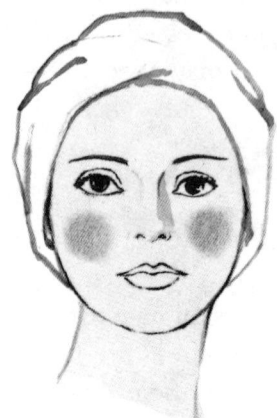

Round

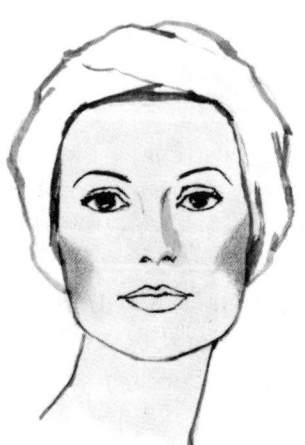

Square

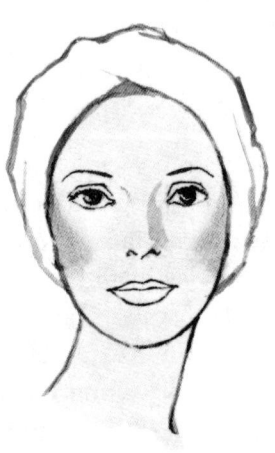

Oval

10. Lipstick. Experts agree that older women should wear lipstick a shade stronger than younger women do. Stronger meaning more intense, not darker in color.

Keeping this in mind, here are some of the things to consider in working with your lips:

   a. Lipstick brush? Models usually use a brush. It controls the contour of the lips, which is important to them in close-up photography. If you are comfortable using a brush, you will always have a neat lip line.
   b. Pencil outliner? If you use one, don't use a strong red. A light brown is surprisingly good if the line is kept very thin with a sharply pointed pencil. The reason for a line is usually corrective. Say that if your upper lip is too thin, you can draw a line at the farthest edge of the lip and fill in with your own shade of lipstick, making the lip look larger. Lower lip too big? Bring your foundation over the lip line and draw your line inside the real one. The most important use of line for almost everybody is to *bring the lines of the lower lip up to the corners more sharply than the regular lip line.* Get your lipstick and liner out right now and try it. Look at the pleasant expression it creates. It takes any sad look away. Clowns found this out a long time ago. Older lips may lose their firm line and allow lipstick to bleed into the lines around the mouth. A chalky pencil liner can keep this from happening.
   c. The old indelible lipstick is passé and I guess for good cause, because it was very drying. I mourn it. I haven't bought a lipstick in some time that stays on very well. Recently I gave an older friend of mine a lipstick that I thought was a good color for her. A few months later she gave it back. "It doesn't stay on," she said. I knew she had gone back to one of her old, too-dark indelibles, and was very happy. I hardly blamed her.
   d. Lip gloss. This takes patience and hourly application. It looks very nice, so use it by all means if you have that kind of time.

COLOR:

I am really in trouble here, because I cannot know your skin tone, rouge color, hair color, clothes selection for the day, or your mouth size. But here are some suggestions that may help:
   a. If the mouth is too small or too big or in any other way not pretty, use soft, light colors. Don't play it up, lose it.
   b. Blonds normally need soft, light colors but those may need to be intensified if the skin tone is dark or sallow.
   c. If you are wearing a garment in the purples, oranges, pinks, reds, or peach shades, watch that the lipstick doesn't clash. Earth tones blend with all and don't glare.
   d. Keep your lipstick and rouge in the same color. This can't be done by holding them together. They can turn different colors when thy react to your skin.
   e. I can't stress enough that you keep away from the purple and bluish shades, no matter what your coloring.

There is another feature of makeup that many of you may never have gotten into, and that is corrective makeup. As a model agent I worked mostly with improving the features, with dark and light makeup to hide the bad features and play up the good. Here are a few simple rules to help you with any problems you may have:
   1) Use a light-weight base, three shades lighter than your regular foundation, under your eyes, at the crowfeet, between the eyebrows if you have frown lines, and down the line from the nose to the chin. Blend it into the edges so it doesn't make just a definite streak.
   2) If you have any touch of sag beneath the chin, use a foundation three shades darker all the way to the base of the neck. Don't let the color become obvious. In the summer, with a little tan on your neck, it won't be noticeable, but in the winter you may want to lighten it.
   3) If you have a jutting jaw, use the darker makeup up onto the chin, following the jawbone around. This is particularly a blending problem. Take great pains.

Corrective Makeup

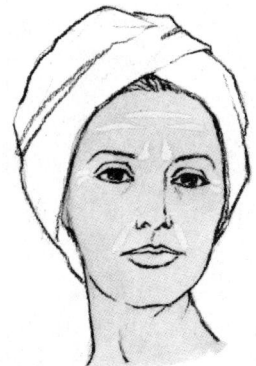

Wrinkles

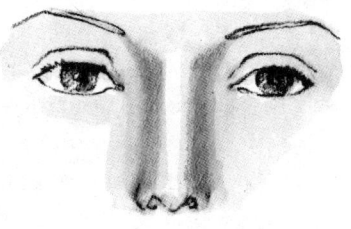

Wide nose

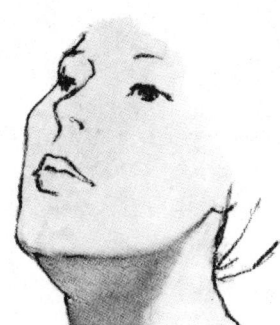

Sagging chin

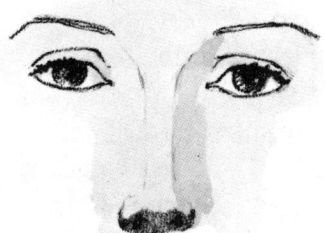

Long nose

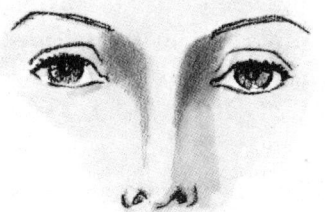

Wide bridge

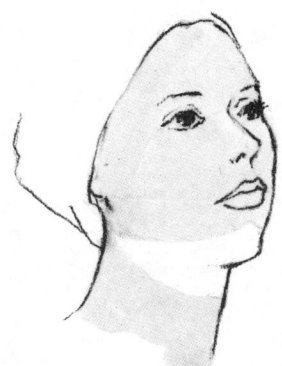

Receeding chin

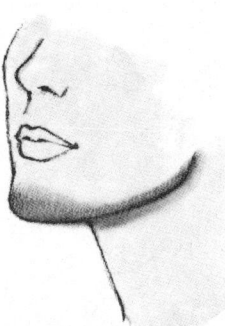

Jutting chin

4) A wide nose? Use your darker makeup on either side and if the bridge is wide, too, carry it all the way up. The bridge of the nose is a beauty spot not noticed by most. It is very feminine and gives the face a delicate look. Now run a light shade down the center of your nose and you may have a thin nose for the first time in your life.
5) If your forehead is too high, use darker makeup at the hairline. Too low, use light.
6) To shorten the nose, darken the tip and blend up onto the nose.
7) A receding chin? Use very light base in a triangle with the point ending at the lower lip. Carry the chinline halfway back the length of the jawbone.

There are many individual structural problems. If you have something you have always hated, remember the theory that light stands out and dark recedes and get to work.

There is only one big "don't." A friend and I were trying to recall the name of someone we had both known. She said, "Oh, you mean 'Early Halloween.'" She was right. Our mutual friend was pretty heavily into the paint pots. Doesn't this describe perfectly some of the women you see on the streets? Some of your friends? I hope not you.

> O wad the power the giftie gie us
> To see oursels as others see us!
> —"To a Louse,"
> by Robert Burns

4
Diet for the Woman with Too Many Pounds

If you have been ten pounds overweight for the past ten years, you are officially obese. How do you like that word *obese*? Doesn't that rock you? The dictionary definition for obese is "extremely fat," from the Latin word "obesus" meaning "grown fat from eating." It may not seem that ten extra pounds is worth the categorizing as "extremely fat," but, as you may have found out, ten pounds and you keep on and on. See the chart on page 56 to determine what your weight should be for your height and age.

Are you ten pounds overweight? Even if you haven't been for ten years, now is the time to do something about it. Those old Romans had the answer to why you have those extra pounds, you know, "grown fat from eating."

Life insurance statistics show us that ten women to one man are overweight in their middle to late years. This is primarily due to menopause, which puts inches on the waist and hips of the majority of women. I don't happen to believe you have to settle for that as an inevitability. You don't wake up in the morning with three extra

DESIRABLE WEIGHTS FOR WOMEN OF AGES 25 AND OVER
Weight in Pounds According to Frame (In Indoor Clothing)

HEIGHT (with shoes on) 2-inch heels		SMALL FRAME	MEDIUM FRAME	LARGE FRAME
Feet	Inches			
4	10	92– 98	96–107	104–119
4	11	94–101	98–110	106–122
5	0	96–104	101–113	109–125
5	1	99–107	104–116	112–128
5	2	102–110	107–119	115–131
5	3	105–113	110–122	118–134
5	4	108–116	113–126	121–138
5	5	111–119	116–130	125–142
5	6	114–123	120–135	129–146
5	7	118–127	124–139	133–150
5	8	122–131	128–143	137–154
5	9	126–135	132–147	141–158
5	10	130–140	136–151	145–163
5	11	134–144	140–155	149–168
6	0	138–148	144–159	153–173

© 1969 Metropolitan Life Insurance Company

inches on your waistline. It creeps up on you gradually, in plenty of time to catch it at the first sign and do something about it with exercise and a change in your eating habits. If it is already too late, it will just take a little longer.

I am sure your doctor has been encouraging you to lose weight for some time. I sometimes wish doctors would come right out with it: "Lose weight or you are laying yourself wide open to a heart attack," for instance. That might help curb your appetite a little. When you are over thirty-five years old, your life expectancy decreases 1 percent for every pound you are overweight. Why? Because excessive pounds can cause trouble with the kidneys, the pancreas, the heart, and the circulatory system. According to Dr. Joan Gomez in her book *How Not to Die Young*, excessive weight can be "as far-reaching as cancer."

In this book I am concerned with your looking and feeling better. I want you to lose weight so you can wear your clothes better (with your new-found waistline). I want you to walk better. Extra weight makes your body too cumbersome to move with agility and grace. I want you to think more positively about yourself—in getting that dress size down, in tightening that belt.

Pride and self-esteem won't be of much value to you if you have succumbed to the physical problems that can result from carrying too many extra pounds.

Cardiovascular diseases* are the first on all lists of mortality rates compiled in the United States and in most European countries. Overweight is unanimously considered the primary contributing factor.

The pancreas, when overworked from too many carbohydrates (primarily refined sugars), will rebel and diabetes will result. Of course, all middle-aged overweights are not diabetics, but the possibility exists.

If your kidneys are overworked, they can cause plenty of trouble. One-quarter of the blood in your system goes through your kidneys for cleansing. A disfunction or infection is no fun.

So to retain your health through your later years, let's start now to get rid of some pounds. Let's get our doctor's okay to do this, however. If you have any chronic diseases or any health problems, make sure that the following suggestions for eating are not contrary to anything your doctor has recommended.

How many full-length mirrors do you have in your house? Well, get one if there are none. You can get a cheap one in most discount stores, sometimes even one with a little frame. Put it in a place that you pass all the time at home. I really mean this. There is no better way to inspire yourself to lose weight than to watch those hips bounce every time you go by the mirror. If you are so used to those hips that they don't faze you anymore, take off your clothes. Where is that girlish figure now, with all the girdles and bras removed? Jump up and down. Are you ready for a diet?

* Cardiovascular diseases: Relating to the heart and blood vessels.

"My husband loves me the way I am!" (If you have a husband, you are one out of four if you are over fifty.) He loves you healthy, though, and you had better convince him that a few pounds removed might give him a wife for a few years longer. If you lose weight as gradually as I am going to recommend, he won't even notice, except to see that you look younger.

That is the truth. In most cases, you *will* look younger with some pounds off. Your friends and/or fellow-workers will compliment you and envy you. It might even stir *them* to lose some pounds. You will see how this decision to lose weight can start a chain reaction that may save a life. You can be a regular heroine, and beautiful, too!

Are you ready to start yet? The decision has to come from you. I had a friend once whose husband was president of a large corporation. She was heavy, very heavy. One day he offered her a hundred dollars for every pound she lost. If you think she bought a new mink coat with the money, you're mistaken. It wasn't her idea, she felt forced into a move she hadn't decided on for herself, and she never did lose any weight. When I saw her again, ten years later, she still weighed her same 180 pounds.

You've got to want to do it yourself. You've got to have that little screw upstairs turn, so you know the time has come. All right? Let's pick Tuesday for the big day. Then you can have a nice, quiet controlled four days before the temptation-filled weekend. Four days to kind of organize yourself, to find where you are going to start with my ten "do's" and ten "don't's" for better eating.

How much do you want to lose? I have had many overweight women apply for modeling jobs. How much they should lose was always the first question. I never said thirty pounds. I said, "Lose five pounds and come back and see me." If they were sincere and lost the first five pounds, the next five were easier, and so on, until some real beauties emerged thirty pounds later.

So let's try this for ourselves. Let's start this Tuesday to lose five pounds. There are so many books and articles with special weight-losing diets (some crazy) that you could be reading for a year. I did.

Here is my own Rule of Ten "do's" and "don't's," which has worked successfully for my models and for me.

Ten "do's" for your new eating life:

1. Get a small calorie-counting booklet at any bookstore, one that is small enough to fit into your purse. Keep it with you when you are confronted with restaurant menus. You won't have to do this for long, because you will soon learn what to avoid. Add to this a small notebook, preferably lined and with at least two columns. Keep track of what you eat, with the calorie count listed beside it. You may want to do this at the end of the day, or you may be able to do it at the end of each meal. However you do it, add it up at the end of the day. Some days you will be over your allotted 1,500 calories, and some days you will be proud to be under that count. This makes calorie counting a game with yourself and adds a little fun and challenge to the project.

2. Eat plenty of protein. It is a medical fact that as the body ages the need for protein increases. It is also true that your calorie requirements are reduced. So your 1,500 calories should be high in protein. That won't be so hard when you take a look at the foods available to you. They are: meats, fish, poultry, brewers' yeast, whole grains, seeds, nuts, milk and milk products (cheese, yogurt), legumes (beans, dried peas, lentils), and eggs. There are small amounts of protein in fruits and vegetables.

3. Exercise. It helps your heart action and circulation and can help you lose inches where you need it the most. More about this later—a *lot* more.

4. Keep your food buying down and your refrigerator sparse so you can't find anything interesting to eat in your frantic moments. I just want to say here that I have found this a most valuable deterrent. With none of these succulent little tidbits around, temptation is removed. If you have teen-agers around ignore this, or stiffen your backbone.

5. Lay your fork down several times while you are eating. You will find that you chew more slowly and, lo and behold, you will discover that you are tasting your food more and eating less. More people rush their food over their taste buds so fast they don't get the most out of its flavor. Watch some of your neighboring diners the next time you are in a restaurant. The shoveling of food into mouths will disgust you. Studies have shown that the pathologically overweight don't taste their food very much at all. The act of eating itself satisfies their psychological needs.

6. Eat breakfast! As much as doctors and nutritionists preach, there are many, many people in the business world and elsewhere who do not have anything to start their day but a cup of coffee.

Nutritionists say that you should eat more meals for a healthful reducing regime—starting with breakfast. If what you are after is health and beauty, let's face the physical facts. Blood sugar in your body drops during the morning in proportion to the amount of protein eaten at breakfast. If there is no food, the blood sugar at noon is very low, producing fatigue and a droopy, unbeautiful look. Protein is what you need for a zippier morning, so if you add a little wheat germ (available at any grocery store) to your cereals, eat an egg at least three times a week, eat whole-grain toast, and maybe add a few nuts or seeds to your cereals, you will have a better morning. My son licked the midmorning blahs by eating liver in the morning. Try it, it's delicious.

But if you can't face solid food, try a small glass of milk. Next day get a little bigger glass. The next day add two tablespoons of non-instant powdered milk and shake it up. Got that down? Next day, add a raw egg to the mixture and shake it up. Presto! You have your protein for maintaining you for a good morning's work, and it slides down easily.

CALORIES:

1 cup skim milk	90
2 tbs. noninstant powdered milk	109
1 egg	80
	279 = less than ⅓ of your daily 1,500 calories

7. Eat something from each of the four basic foods each day. They are:
1. Milk and cheese
2. Meat, poultry, fish, eggs
3. Vegetables and fruits
4. Cereals and breads

a. Note that skim milk, which is strong in protein, vitamins and minerals, is only 90 calories a cup. Cottage cheese is high in nutrition and low in calories, 1 ounce equals 25 calories.

1 cup sour cream	485 calories
1 cup skim milk yogurt	150 calories

I have found that yogurt can be used in cooking and salads without anyone knowing the difference. Cucumbers and yogurt are indeed a treat. Try prune whip with yogurt. I put yogurt in milk and shake it up. Linda Clark includes it in the list of "wonder foods" in her book *Stay Young Longer*.

Why all the fuss about yogurt? In the European countries, where it is most often eaten, people seem to live longer (many live to over a hundred), and with more energy. This is certainly a good thought to hold onto when planning your next menu. The action of the yogurt destroys the putrefactive bacteria, which in simple terms aids your digestion and helps to prevent constipation. I can vouch for that. Whether or not it will help me to live to be a hundred remains to be seen.

b. Meats, fish, poultry, and eggs are not likely to be left out of a diet in this high-meat-consuming nation. Just make sure you take off the fat first. Make sure you have meat of some food value, though. Pressed lunch meats and hot dogs don't give you much food for your money. One-eighth inch slice of bologna has 68 calories . . . 68 calories just to put something in your stomach? One hot dog has 182 calories. A 60-gram hot dog contains 7.4 grams of protein, 8 percent, and not much else in food value. That is hardly worth all those calories, do you think?

c. The whole fruit and vegetable family combined takes in a lot of territory. For instance, there are root vegetables, leafy vegetables, shoots, seed vegetables, and pods. Th most important in vitamin content are the leafy, but don't forget the others. The following list will show you some to avoid in your next few months of trying to lose weight.

These are all fresh-cooked vegetables, but the frozen equivalents are not much different in food value. Given a choice, this will give an idea of where you can knock off calories in seemingly innocent vegetables:

1 cup green peas = 115 cal.	1 cup green beans = 32 cal.
1 cup lima beans = 190 cal.	1 cup carrots = 44 cal.
1 cup beets = 55 cal.	1 cup cauliflower = 20 cal.
1 cup winter squash = 72 cal.	1 cup summer squash = 30 cal.
1 cup mixed vegetables = 114 cal.	1 cup spinach = 40 cal.
1 baked sweet potato = 155 cal.	1 baked white potato = 140 cal.

The list can go on and on.

Fruits are equally numerous. The most important group is citrous. The vitamin count is a little higher in oranges than in grapefruit, but so is the calorie count. Keep a little heavier on grapefruit consumption and save the calories. If you have been drinking prune juice, forget it; it has 200 calories a cup, compared to 120 for orange juice and 100 for grapefruit juice.

All the other fruits are good, and necessary, but watch the sweetened syrup in the canned ones. It shoots the calorie count way up and doesn't add anything to the food value of the fruit.

d. By now you should not be wasting your calories on white bread when wheat breads have twice the protein, less calories, and many more nutrients. There are many combinations of whole grains in breads to please your tastes. Switch around and you'll get a change in nutritious content and more fun.

Prepared cereals can be pretty high in calories because they contain sweeteners. The granola types have more nutrition but have four to five times the calorie content. Even if you are used to eating cereal for breakfast, try adding another one of Linda Clark's "wonder foods," wheat germ. It is high in the B vitamins and some minerals and tastes good. It contains 38 calories per teaspoonful and, sprinkled on lots of things including salads, adds greatly to our nutrition for the day without adding greatly to our calories. I add wheat germ to hamburgers, meat loaf, peanut butter (the unhomogenized kind with the natural oil on top). You can let your imagination run wild.

8. Do eat your meat and vegetables without folderols. No gravies or sauces for the meats. This will be a tough go for those of you who have formed lifelong habits of using catsup and chili sauce on everything. I find the gravy/sauce habit especially prevalent in southern cooking. I blame that on the drying of most meats by overcooking, which makes them hard to eat without a lubricant. When you do stop using your favorite sauce, you will soon find a taste in your meat that you hadn't known was there. This is especially true of vegetables. When they have been cooked in a small amount of water, quickly, so they retain a crisper texture, they have a sweetness that doesn't require a lot of added flavors, butter, or margarine. You are cutting out calories that are certainly not needed, which you will soon not miss.

9. Do be aware of using your food as a reward. Most of us do this without realizing it. If you are conscious of this reason for eating some of the reward foods, it will be a little easier to control this.

When you were a little girl you got a lollipop when you were good. This started with the parent doling out the treat. Most of us have incorporated this habit into our own lives, becoming our own monitors—with candy bars, cookies, or martinis when we are tired or mad at the world. How many times have you heard, "I deserve a drink tonight after what I went through today"?

The reward we have to switch our minds to is a thinner, longer, healthier, and more beautiful life.

It's hard. You won't always win. I don't. I had a great piece of chocolate cake the other day and it didn't kill me. Until you get used to this new way of eating, don't get hemmed in so you can't have *anything* you want. I do not hold with the rigid-type diets that frustrate you into quitting after a few weeks.

Stop using sugar in your coffee; then cut out the fancy desserts; lead up to cutting out that midmorning snack of heaven knows what. You'll be surprised how your calorie notebook will help you. Seeing those figures on paper is a real stopper. What you will develop, if you take it easy and let each improvement become permanent, is a new chain of thought about food that will be with you for the rest of your life.

10. And the last do. Do plan your meals ahead. As you get older, fewer new cells are formed in your body. It is absolutely essential to keep your remaining cells at the peak of health. They are not being replaced as they were when you were twenty. Take good care of them with a planned diet that includes foods from the four basic groups we have just read about in rule 7. I really mean that, unless you think about this, plan for it, and shop for it, you can find yourself eating anything that is handy.

Everyone's approach will be different. I avoid regimentation, so I keep a subconscious awareness of what I am eating. This won't work for everyone. Maybe in your notebook you will want to check off the four basics every day to see that you haven't missed any. The next day you will plan better, until your awareness of each food becomes automatic.

To help you in your planning, there are many excellent recipes and menus for the dieter. The following list of books leans heavily to good nutrition: Gaylord Hauser, *Mirror, Mirror, on the Wall;* Adelle Davis, *Let's Cook It Right;* Ellen Buckman Ewald, *Recipes for a Small Planet* (try this one for some vey interesting and tasty meatless meals); Ann Gold and Sara Welles Briller, *The Diet Watcher's Gourmet Cookbook;* Eileen Ford, *A More Beautiful You in 21 Days;* Beatriz-Marie Proda, *200 Really Great Natural Food Recipes.*

There are many more, but be sure that they encompass complete nutrition if you get into them.

When you really have yourself in the diet groove, don't retract. Don't give up in a few weeks. The pounds you lost will be right back, and all this effort will be lost. Don't *start* if you can't keep it up. The diet yo-yo's are a well-recognized group. They are either just starting or have just fallen off of a diet. This kind of procedure is not for us. It puts an added strain on the heart.

How long will it take you to attain any permanent weight reduction? This is difficult to answer, since our metabolisms are all so different.

What is metabolism? It is "the process by which foods are transformed into basic elements which can be used by the body for energy and growth."

To lose the first five pounds, don't be disappointed if it takes a month. You want this weight to stay off permanently if you want to live to be a hundred. Crash diets don't keep the weight off and are age-adding. They are not rounded diets and are depriving you of your much-needed nutrition. You will sag, look strained, and miss the whole point of losing weight: to make you more beautiful.

Let me warn you that you will encounter plateaus of no loss for several days sometimes. Then, boom, you'll drop two pounds. Just keep your notebook in hand and keep going. There is a variety of opinion in dieting circles as to when you should weigh yourself—once a week, once every two weeks. I like to weigh every day. It keeps my mind on what I am attempting to do. It's bad on those no-loss days, but is it thrilling when you look down and see those two pounds gone!

Before we go on to my ten "don't's" for diet eating, I want you to ask yourself one question. "Why do I overeat?" Is it because you just eat the same old things you have always eaten, in the same amounts, the same food your mother used to cook? You won't when you get those calories down on paper. Or do you say to yourself secretly, "I am sure it is my glands." As the kids say, this is a cop out. The small number of glandular patients, compared to the large number of overweight people, doesn't bear out this excuse. If you really want to know, however, you certainly should see your doctor.

Is it that you think you need sugar for energy? You tire easily and that midmorning coke or midafternoon candy bar gives you a lift? It could also be from boredom and need for reward, couldn't it?

This kind of quick energy won't get you far, not as far as a handful of nuts or sunflower seeds (another "wonder" food). They contain protein and the energy from protein is far more sustaining.

Maybe your willpower is lacking.

Frank J. Bringe, in his fine book *Think Yourself Thin*, says that human beings have the ability to control fixed habits. Animals do not. According to him, you can easily stop eating bread at every meal if you want to. Now this seems pretty obvious. The ability to control fixed habits requires a motive, like walking to work in a driving snowstorm to get to work on time. Willpower, the drive that is controlled by the motive, gets you through.

On the negative side, it is harder. Willpower must move us to a "not doing." "Don't eat that cake." "No sugar, thank you." Your motive has to dig deep into your subconscious, because it is not an immediate reward. Your motive is your own important health—and ultimately your life-span.

Have you found that your eating is really uncontrollable?

Food can be a real psychological problem that is complicated and highly emotional. *Think Yourself Thin* might be of some help to you if you are facing this problem. It presents different types of problem eaters and offers suggestions for help that are very realistic. It is available in paperback in most bookstores or it can be ordered.

Ready for more?

Here is my Rule of Ten Don't's for a thinner, more beautiful you:

1. Cut down on all your carbohydrates, sugar, and starch. No sugar in your coffee or tea. One teaspoon of sugar is 52 calories, times 3 cups a day, is 156 calories you could utilize in a day for more useful food values.

"Food value" means "contains nutrients."

"Nutrients" means "containing vitamins, minerals, and proteins necessary for the bodily functions."

These habits are hard to break. I was lucky, because it was a point of distinction in my college crowd not to use sugar, so I got onto the right foot early. Social motivation when you are young can cure you of anything—or get you into anything.

Maybe you are the clean break type who can give up anything you set your mind to. If not, try the slow cutback method. One-half teaspoon instead of a whole one.

Small portions of potatoes, pasta, and bread must be watched and eaten with reservations, but never eat starch at *all three meals.*

Desserts are out except for fresh fruits, which you need. Keep track of their calorie count, as some are much higher than others. Canned fruit is acceptable, but don't eat the syrup. Better still, get the unsweetened. They are on the shelves in the diet-food sections of most grocery stores.

2. Don't eat the fat on meats, or fatty meats. This includes steaks for awhile, which are heavily marbled with fats. This is certainly contrary to the steak and grapefruit diets that were so popular a while back.

Absolutely no hamburger unless you have the butcher grind you especially lean meat.

Fish is best.

Veal is better than beef, if all the fat is cut off.

Lamb is all right, if all the fat is cut off.

Pork is the least desirable, but if eaten cut off fat.

Chicken is fine, but do not eat the skin.

3. Don't add salt at the table. Salt causes water retention, which keeps weight on the scales. You can actually lose weight from the fatty areas of the body and still show more weight on the scales. Diuretics are foolers and do no lasting good. A model I know used to take diuretics just before every fashion show so she could fit into the clothes. The next day she was back to bloat.

4. Don't eat "empty calories." They are called various picturesque names like "junk," "foolish," or "naked." They are self-explanatory, of course, meaning "containing no food value." I guess the explicitness of the name made me see them for what they really were and helped me to stop eating them. It made me stop and think about everything else I ate. Was it just "junk" or was it doing something for me?

Here are some empty calorie foods: Doughnuts, sweet rolls,

coffee cake, candy bars, cake, soft drinks (even low-cal), potato chips, French fries.

"How do I eat that hamburger without French fries?" When you get your mind adjusted to some of your diet excesses, you will soon find the will to do without them. Of course you tell the waiter to leave them off your plate, so they are not sitting there staring at you.

How do you have your morning coffee without that sweet roll? Let the number 275 ring loud and clear in your head: 275 calories for a Danish? That is one-sixteenth of your 1,500 calories shot, with lunch and dinner yet to come.

This is the thinking that you will be doing as I have, and it works.

5. Don't snack. Don't just throw food into your mouth from boredom or nervous tension. It's more than likely to be from the "empty calories" list. But maybe you are not doing well on a diet where you eat three meals a day. Adelle Davis recommends eating smaller meals and eating more often. I like this myself some days, when nothing seems to fill me up. If you plan what you are going to eat and make a meal of each of the four foods that count in nutrition, *and* watch the calories, why not?

Don Gerraud has written a book called *One Bowl,* in which he recommends just that. All your food in one bowl, and eaten whenever you are hungry, and forgetting the time of day. Even if the others in your family are at the table, he thinks you eat with more concentration and digest better without any disturbing conversation if you take your bowl to another part of the house.

Well, I guess I have sat at tables occasionally that were pretty raucous. My digestion must have suffered; but then there were the good times that must have stimulated it.

6. Don't eat everything on your plate. If you are in a restaurant, or not at home where you can control the portions, don't just eat it because it is there. You may think you are wasting food, but I can't see how that food can be any asset when it is turning into fat on you. The old clean-your-plate thinking stems from childhood, of course. My mother used to make me eat everything she gave me because of the starving Armenians. I didn't know why the Armenians were starving until many years and much history later. One theory on the cause for superfat people stems from their early years with food-pushing mothers.

7. Don't take diet pills. Most doctors won't prescribe them, but if you should talk yours into some remember that they will only benefit you while you are taking them. Then you must fall right back on your own self-discipline. Permanent weight loss can only come from eating the correct foods over a period of time.

8. Don't use diet formulas more than once a day. That is, any brand of the liquid canned food supplements. They have adequate food value, but they cannot take the place of foodstuffs with the equivalent calorie count. To eat regular foods is much more rewarding psychologically and they are needed for body functions.

9. Don't drink alcohol. These are wasted words, I know, when you are in certain social situations. Just remember that the calories are high, with no food values received.

Some of the horrible facts about the calorie count in cocktails:

Bloody Mary: 130
Martini: 140
Old Fashioned: 179
Whiskey Sour: 175
Manhattan: 164
Wines are better (3½ to 4 oz.):
    Champagne: 84
    Red wine: 81
    White wine: 74
    Dessert wine: 140
Beer (8 oz.): 114

One of the problems with alcohol is that it stimulates the appetite. When this happens at the same time that your defenses are down, what do you suppose happens? You are right, you overeat.

It is best to forego the nightly cocktail, if you are used to one, until you lose a few pounds. By this I mean that the first few weeks are the least rewarding and you really have to pare down to the bone to get started losing. After that, it is easier.

10. Don't forget to consult your doctor before starting on a program for a very large weight loss. I would say over fifteen pounds would be the most you should plan without getting an okay from him, regardless of your health.

With these twenty thoughts in mind, let us go on to the next chapter. This one will help you build your health while you are taking off pounds.

Keep your notebook and calorie counter in hand. Count every day.

Bibliography

Atkins, Robert. *Dr. Atkins' Diet Revolution.* New York: Bantam, 1973.
Bruno, Frank J. *Think Yourself Thin.* Plainview, N.Y.: Nash, 1972.
Cantor, Alfred. *Dr. Cantor's Longevity Diet.* New York: Award Books, 1967.
Clark, Linda. *Stay Young Longer.* New York: Pyramid Communications, Inc., 1974.
Crenshaw, Mary Ann. *Super Beauty.* New York: David McKay, 1974.
Davis, Adelle. *Let's Cook It Right.* New York: New American Library, 1970.
Ewald, Ellen Buckman. *Recipes for a Small Planet.* New York: Ballantine Books, 1973.
Ford, Eileen. *A More Beautiful You in 21 Days.* New York: Simon & Schuster, 1973.
Gerard, Don. *One Bowl.* New York: Random House, 1974.
Gold, Ann and Briller, Sara Welles. *The Diet Watcher's Gourmet Cookbook.* New York: Grosset & Dunlap, 1969.
Gomez, Joan. *How Not to Die Young.* New York: Pocket Books, 1973.
Hauser, Gaylord. *Mirror, Mirror, on the Wall.* Greenwich, Conn.: Fawcett, Crest Books, 1961.
Jameson, Gardner, and Elliott Williams. *The Drinking Man's Diet & Cookbook.* New York: Bantam Books, 1973.

Lappe, Frances Moor. *Diet for a Small Planet*. New York: Ballantine Books, 1971.
Prada, Beatriz-Marie. *200 Really Great Natural Food Recipes*. New York: Ballantine, 1972.
Serino, G. S. *Reducing After 40*. Philadelphia: Auerbach Publishers, 1971.

5
Vitamins to Keep You Healthy

Izaak Walton said, "Look to your health and if you have it, praise God, and value it next to your conscience: for health is the second blessing we mortals are capable of; a blessing money cannot buy." Today, we mortals are more fortunate, since we can buy a whole lot of health from any vitamin shelf.

There is no point in losing weight just to look pale and haggard. Our aim is to look as beautiful as we possibly can, using the good judgment we should have acquired by now. So let us look for a minute at what makes up these bodies of ours. I have already pointed out that, as we get older, our cells do not replenish themselves as quickly as when we were younger. All living things—plants, animals, and humans—are the sum total of their cells. If there are damaged or less than healthy cells in any part of our body, there is trouble. Our responsibility is to give those cells the best foods possible and supplement them from the vitamin shelves. There are forty requirements for the good health of our cells, which must be supplied by these foods and food supplements.*

* Food supplements: vitamins and minerals.

Vitamins interact with one another and cannot be tested like a medicine, so laboratory testing has been slow. Add to that the problem that deficiencies cannot be tested on humans because of the danger to lives; hence their exact effect on the human body has been difficult to prove. Even though testing with animals has brought to light many problems caused by deficiencies, these clinical tests are not considered conclusive. This has hampered the progress of vitamin research, but even so the Department of Health, Education and Welfare has changed some of its ratings to: "The need in human nutrition has been established but the minimum daily requirement has not been established." This recognition of need is a step forward from the previous rating of: "The need has not been established." The rating I am going to give you in this chapter is the RDR: Recommended Daily Requirement, established by the Department of Health, Education and Welfare.

Here is a list of body requirements and their best sources in available foods. It reads like a broken record. You will see our old friends from the last chapter and Linda Clark's "wonder foods" all over the place. The foods listed are the best-known sources for the given vitamins but are available in lesser amounts in other foods.

1. Protein. The need for protein in the aging cell is greatly accelerated, because the aging cell breaks down faster and does not replace itself as frequently as the younger cells. Protein is the builder of cells. It is involved with the amino acids* in the digestive processes. Because there are eight amino acids and because they are not all present in equal quantities in every protein, don't go out and eat five lamb chops and think your are getting your protein for the day. When they are not all present in one meal, the use your body gets from the protein is only a percentage. When you read the term "complete protein," it means having all the amino acids in the right proportion.

Frances Moore Lappe, in her book *Diet for a Small Planet*, tells the whole story in charts. It is fascinating to see what proteins are best combined to effect the most spectacular improvements in you. For

---
* Amino acids: the product of protein metabolism.

instance, milk added to almost any other protein adds considerably to the usable protein in your meal. Unless you want to make a study of the combinations in the charts, here is a list of the best proteins and you can remember that combinations are better than one alone.

PROTEIN FOODS:

Eggs
Milk and milk products
Meats (liver, kidney, heart)
Muscle meats (steaks, etc.)
Fish
Fowl
Legumes
Beans
Nuts
Whole grains
Seeds
Soy beans and products

2. **Carbohydrates.** Dr. Roger Williams, in his book *Nutrition Against Disease*, states that "the most serious nutrition habit is excess sugar consumption." Refined sugar is a food with no food value, no nutrition, and it goes into your body as fat. And yet Americans consume millions of tons every year. This has been my weakness. Sheer willpower kept me away from gooey desserts and candy bars—well, not altogether. I have been saved by my shift to a high protein diet. Nutritionists say this is a normal result of better eating habits; that sugar craving is the result of a dietary deficiency.

SUGAR:

    a. Overstimulates the production of insulin (leading to diabetes?).
    b. Interferes with the absorption of protein, calcium, and other minerals.

    c. Retards the growth of needed intestinal bacteria.
    d. Takes your appetite from other more nutritious foods.
    e. Goes into fat.

Other carbohydrates are necessary and should not be avoided. Watch their natural sugar content for high calorie count, however. They are:

    Root vegetables
    Whole grain cereals
    Fresh fruits and juices

3. Fats. There are three fatty acids in vegetable oils: lioleic, linolenic, and andochronic. These are very important after you reach certain years. They are important to the digestion and are even used, according to one aging theory, as a rejuvenator.

The commercially produced oils in your supermarket have lost these three important acids through heat processing but the "cold-pressed," "mechanically-pressed" or "hard-pressed" have not. Look on the labels. They are more expensive, but I am convinced that the extra money spent is doing me some good. Of course, any oil you buy should be polyunsaturated. Some nutritionists hold with safflower oil, some with peanut, some with corn; and there are combinations, too. I go for the combinations when I can find them, just in case.

With all the publicity on polyunsaturates, the reason for using them is no news to you, I am sure. Saturated fats produce cholesterol. This leaves fatty deposits in the arteries, slowing down the flow of blood. It causes all kinds of problems, the most common being heart trouble and arteriosclerosis.

Dr. Alfred Cantor, in his book *Dr. Cantor's Longevity Diet,* would have us take one ounce of polyunsaturated oil three times a day. This contains 750 calories. Most other nutritionists agree that oil should be in the diet and find two tablespoons (250 calories) to be adequate. This is easier on the calorie watcher, because it can be added to your salad oils and used in cooking. I up my intake a little, because the older you get the more oil you need, as Dr. Cantor points out.

Polyunsaturated oils are found in:

> Salad dressings (look at labels)
> Mayonnaise (look at labels)
> Nuts
> Sunflower seeds (and others)
> Avocados
> Unhydrogenated peanut butter
> Salad oils

If this seems a lot to absorb all at once, read it again at a later date. There's no fun in being beautiful unless you have good health.

Vitamins

Vitamins in foods are a relatively new discovery. James Lind, back in 1747, who fed English sailors limes to prevent scurvey, did not know it was vitamin C that was doing the trick. Even today doctors are given very short training in nutrition. They are taught to cure disease. It took the nutritionists to come along and teach us how to prevent it.

VITAMIN A

Some authorities believe that there is a widespread deficiency of Vitamin A in our diets.

In the list of 108 faulty body conditions included at the end of this chapter, it appears as having helped twenty-one of them. It first became noted as being helpful in night blindness. It is now considered generally beneficial to the eyes. It is good for the skin, the mucous membrane, even leading into the lungs. It's action is to soften the tissues.

Disagreement over dosage is considerable. It is a fat-soluble vitamin that is stored in the body, and overdosage over a lengthy period can produce toxicity. The controversy comes over how much, and over what period of time, it will cause the toxicity. The Food and Drug Administration has limited the individual daily intake to 4,000 USP units.* Nutritionists give examples of 100,000 to 500,000 units having been tolerated without problems. The American Medical Association says not more than 50,000. Dosage in most multivitamin tablets runs above the 4,000 and without conflict with the regulations. Three to five times the RDR** on any vitamin allowed if it is labeled "therapeutic" dosage.

Dosage: 4,000 USP, RDR

Must be taken with vitamin D for maximum usage in the body.

Foods containing vitamin A:

Cream
Whole milk
Eggs
Liver
Yellow vegetables
Green vegetables
Fruits
Tomatoes

THE B VITAMINS

The B vitamins are a complicated group of ten vitamins, all necessary for our good health. They are needed in proportions according to the individual needs and must be taken together in some cases. I have indicated that in the dosage when it is necessary. Since our individual needs vary so considerably, how do we know how much and what to take? The simplest solution for the average person who just wants everyday good health insurance is to take a B-Complex formula. The next time you buy one, get another brand, then another

* USP units: United States Pharmacopoeia unit of measure

** RDR: Recommended daily requirement.

after that. They can vary widely in their formulas, so a change can insure you against any deficiencies.

You may want to add other Bs individually as you find the use for each that fits a personal problem. I do.

B-1, Thiamine

Most necessary for muscle coordination. This makes it more valuable to the older citizen where this can be a problem. Must be taken if you drink alcohol because alcohol keeps the body from utilizing thiamine. Martin Ebon says facetiously, in his book *Which Vitamins Do You Need,* that every bottle containing alcohol should read "Enriched with Vitamin B-1."

Dosage: RDR—1.5 mg.* Martin Ebon says 3 mg and Adelle Davis says 2 mg. It can be bought in 50 mg tablets and at least one B-Complex contains 50 mg.

I should point out here that water-soluble vitamins can be taken in large quantities without harm, since they are excreted. The only harm they can do is to your pocketbook. There has been a lot said and written about vitamin freaks and their mad consumption beyond all possible need. Since the decision is yours to make, let your good judgment and good health pattern make the choice of amounts.

B-2, Riboflavin

Research has shown that a deficiency of this vitamin can cause anemia, sore lips, pucker lines around the mouth, ulcers, slow healing, and eye problems. This doesn't mean that you are about to fall victim to all of those if you are slightly low in riboflavin. These are problems that have been induced in laboratory situations by extreme deficiencies. We must translate these findings to our own use and conclude that adequate dosage will prevent any of these troubles.

Dosage: RDR—1.7 mg; Martin Ebon—3 mg, Adelle Davis, 3 mg. One B-Complex has 50 mg.

---

* Mg is milligrams and is the most common measure of weight in vitamin dosage. It is 1/1,000th of a gram.

B-3, Niacin

As in the other Bs, you will have to determine your own need. It is noticeable if there is trouble in visual perception, sore tongue, diarrhea, and certain skin pigmentations and has been used in the treatment of iron-deficient anemia and arthritis.

It is called the "blood vessel dilator" and will cause a flushing of the skin unless used as niacinamide. Because of the dilating action, it is used in treating the elderly for mental confusion, and in Canada there is a clinic that is showing good results in treatment for schizophrenia, used together with inositol.

Dosage: RDR—20 mg. Considered low by most. Many recommended 100 mg. One B-Complex formula has 25 mg.

B-12, Cyanocobalamin

Lack of this vitamin causes pernicious anemia, old-age syndromes, heart diseases, poor circulation, asthma, and certain eye disorders. A long time ago I had a friend who held a very important position in the business world until she was seventy-five. Every week she got her B-12 shot. She was quite ahead of her day with a very aware doctor. Let your conscience be your guide.

Dosage: RDR—6 mcg*, B-Complex formula, 100 mcg. Should always be taken with folic acid.

Pantothenic acid, a B vitamin

This is found in all the cells in the body and therefore needed in all of the body functions. It is involved with all the other vitamins to such an extent that it has been hard to separate in the laboratory. However, some testing has shown deficiencies to cause abdominal pain and emotional upsets. It is called the "antistress vitamin" and appears thirty times in my list of 108 body troubles and their vitamin needs.

Dosage: RDR—10 mg; Martin Ebon—20 mg. Can be bought in tablets of 100, 200, and 500 mg.

*Mcg: microgram, 1/1,000th of a milligram.

B-6 Pyridoxine

An important link in the B family. It reduces water retention, especially interesting to you dieters. For "The Pill" users, it reduces leg cramps and other side effects. It controls nausea, hair loss, diarrhea, eczema, and arteriosclerosis. Possibly because it controls the xanthurenic acid in the system, it may help to prevent diabetes. It is particularly needed with a high protein diet, and that's me.

Dosage: DRD—2 mg. Considered very low. One multiple vitamin, 100 mg.

Inositol, a B vitamin

Found in the cells of the heart, eye, brain, making it seemingly necessary for the good functioning of these parts of the body. Experiments have shown a deficiency to cause baldness. Inconclusive experiments have shown it to resist cirrhosis of the liver. It's most important function for us is that it is necessary in the manufacturing of lecithin in our bodies. We will hear more about lecithin shortly, so let it suffice that it keeps our arteries open.

Dosage: RDR—not available. Martin Ebon says 100 mg. One B-Complex has 4.8 mg.

Choline, a B vitamin

It is known for its part in muscle action. It is an important ingredient in the fluid that connects the nerve that signals the muscle action. A deficiency can cause muscles to respond slowly or not at all. It affects the blood pressure, the metabolism of fat and is helpful to the kidneys and the liver.

Dosage: RDR—not available. Martin Ebon says 100 mg. One B-Complex has 3.9 mg.

Folic Acid, a B vitamin

It is helpful in the absorption of food. A deficiency can cause a special type of anemia (megaloblastic). It is needed for the function of other vitamins, such as A, D, E, and K. B-12 and folic acid must be taken together for the best use of both. It is limited in dosage by the

FDA because too much of it in the system makes a type of anemia hard to diagnose.

Dosage: RDR—0.4 mg. Must be taken with B-12.

PABA, a B vitamin (Para aminobenzoic acid)

Can be used externally for the prevention of sunburn. It is used in helping with some types of eczema and skin pigmentation problems and can be taken internally. It helps prevent gray hair. Use the lotion or cream for sun protection and save yourself the dried-prune look of some of your Floridian friends.

Dosage: RDR not available.

These are the B vitamins. They are numerous, necessary, and it's up to you to arrive at the ones that are most needed by your system beyond a good B-Complex, if any.

B vitamins are found in:

Brewer's yeast	Milk
Torula yeast	Cheese
Whole grains	Lentils
Liver	Green vegetables
Fish	Soy beans
Lean meats	Wheat germ
Poultry	Potatoes

Additional sources for folic acid:

Oranges
Grapefruit
Lemons

VITAMIN E

To best understand the action of vitamin E in the body, I will quote from Dr. Evan Shute, who was kind enough to see me in his clinic in London, Ontario. He explains that "our bodies make better use of available oxygen with the addition of vitamin E." Dr. Shute and his brother, Dr. Wilfred Shute, pioneered the use of vitamin E to prevent and cure problems of the circulatory system over a period of thirty-five years.

Here is a list of problems that they worked with:

1. Angina pectoris: pain in the chest due to a narrowing of arteries that supply blood to the heart muscles.
2. Increasing exercise tolerance.
3. Reducing blood clots.
4. Peripheral vascular diseases: those that limit the blood supply to the legs, feet, arms, and hands. Very important in later years.
5. Reducing difficulties in breathing.
6. Phlebitis: a clot restricting the flow of blood.
7. Varicose veins.
8. Embolism: blood clots that disintegrate after surgery and are carried by the blood stream to the lungs, sometimes fatally.
9. Burns: at the Shute Institute there are slides showing remarkable cures from severe burns, effected without skin grafting. The Institute works with both megadosages and ointments. Ointment is available with vitamin E at any drugstore and is a good thing to keep around the house.
10. Prevention of scar tissue.

Are you impressed? Well, there are still doctors who are not. I heard one on a panel not long ago say of vitamin E: "Oh, just tell them to go eat a hamburger." Luckily that kind of thinking is not prevalent.

Since it is not compatible with iron, mineral oil, and estrogen, vitamin E should be taken ten hours after any of these. It is used up by them, leaving it unavailable to the rest of the body. Polyunsaturated fats also use up E, which has led some nutritionists in the last ten years to theorize that the additional need for E comes directly from the greatly increased consumption of polyunsaturated fats.

Because E reduces the need for oxygen in the cells, there are researchers who find that since the aging process accelerates oxidation, it is retarded by the use of E. This should be of interest to all of us. And since it has been used successfully in the treatment of the heart, the arteries and the slowed-down blood flow to the extremities, I am convinced that this vitamin is for me—and you.

Dosage: RDR—30 IU.* Dr. Wilfred Shute, in his book *Vitamin E for Ailing and Healthy Hearts,* says 200 IU and to make sure the label says alpha tocopheral.

Warning: There are two conditions in which E should not be taken in large doses without a doctor's surveillance: anyone with high blood pressure or anyone who has had rheumatic fever at any time.

Vitamin E is found in:

Wheat germ
Wheat germ oil
Eggs
Fish
Whole wheat
Vegetable oils

Let us pause for breath. This is an awful lot to absorb in one reading. But it will all be there to go back to for reference when you need it. My hope is that you will not read this book from cover to cover like a novel but take each chapter to heart and give it plenty of time and thought. That way, each chapter can surely add something new to your life, something to make you more beautiful inside and out. This chapter is to make you beautiful inside. However, treating those cells kindly is going to show on the outside in better color, skin, and hair texture.

On to more vitamins!

VITAMIN C

The most controversial of them all, not as to the need but as to the amount needed. It all started with Dr. Linus Pauling's book, *Vitamin C and the Common Cold.* His claims for its miraculous cures

---

* IU: International unit.

were challenged by doctors and nutritionists alike. It has been conceded that it cannot be ignored in the treatment for colds. Taking individual differences into account and adding to that the hundred or more viruses that can cause colds, it is no wonder that laboratories have not arrived at the same conclusions. Since it is a body nutrient found in every cell, supplementing your diet each day and accelerating the dosage when you feel cold symptoms can't do any harm. Maybe the bug that is trying to get you will be one that vitamin C will discourage.

Vitamin C is a detoxifying agent and should be taken when you are being dosed with certain toxic drugs. This detoxifying action is good to keep in mind, since one of the theories of aging is the body's slowing down of its ability to get rid of toxic materials. It is also necessary in later years because it protects the adrenal glands under stress. As the glands slow down, C stimulates the secretions.

"Stress," as used by nutritionists, means any condition that harms the body. This can include emotional disturbances, illness, surgery, or any other than normal condition.

Dosage: RDR—60 mg. Under stress conditions, Dr. Pauling goes up to 10,000 mg, and Adelle Davis to 4,000.

Vitamin C is found in:

- Citrus fruits
- Other fruits
- Leafy vegetables
- Broccoli
- Cauliflower
- Tomatoes

VITAMIN D

"The sunshine vitamin." If you live in a climate with continuous sun and don't stay in the house all day, the chances are you won't need to add vitamin D to your diet. But, if you don't get sunshine and don't drink one quart of milk a day, fortified by D, you had better make sure with a supplement. It is important to us because it is necessary in the absorption of calcium. We need calcium to be completely available for our porous bones after menopause, for our "widow's hump," for the bone supporting our teeth and for our teeth.

Dosage: 400 IU. This is limited, because it is oil soluble and remains in the system instead of being excreted, possibly causing toxic effects.

VITAMIN K

Vitamin K is necessary for clotting of the blood. It is formed from intestinal bacteria normally, but antibiotics inhibit the formation. Yogurt can be eaten to bring the action back to normal.

Dosage: No need for supplements.

Vitamin K is found in:

- Green leafy vegetables
- Alfalfa
- Cabbage
- Egg yolks
- Liver

VITAMIN H (Biotin)

This vitamin is helpful in counteracting some allergies. It helps synthesize* fats in the liver. A deficiency can cause eczema, hair loss, and scaly skin.

Dosage: RDR—0.3 mg. It is found in many foods so additional amounts are not required.

Vitamin H is found in:

- Green leafy vegetables
- Liver
- Kidneys
- Meats

*Synthesis: formation of complex substances from a combination of simple substances.

VITAMIN P (Bioflavenoids)

Needed to strengthen the blood vessels to prevent blood clots.
Dosage: Considered adequate in the diet.
Vitamin P is found in:

White skin of oranges
Lemons
Apricots
Grapes

And that's it. This completes the list of known vitamins of any importance. I have tried to point out the help they can offer for aging cells when their use is known. Dosages are indeed in confusion and most nutritionists hesitate to give a one-for-all list. It depends on one's individual needs, which can only be worked out by trial and error on your own.

Minerals

Vitamins do not complete the body requirements. The following minerals will further enlighten you as to what goes on under your skin.

IRON

It is no news to you as a woman that this deficiency causes the commonest type of anemia, resulting in fatigue and headaches. There are few of us who haven't had some degree of anemia at some time or another. This is common because of menstrual loss. It is important in later years for good quality of the blood.

Dosage: RDR—18 mg, considered adequate in the diet if there is no stress condition.

Iron is found in:

Brewer's yeast
Meat
Eggs

Whole grain breads
Cereals
Fruits
Nuts

POTASSIUM

Needed if on a low-salt diet, by diabetics, and if cortizone is being taken. A deficiency of potassium in the adrenal glands can cause a rise in blood pressure. It should be taken when diuretics are taken frequently.

Dosage: Ample is supplied by the diet unless prescribed by a doctor.

Potassium is found in:

Nuts
Meats
Poultry
Whole grains
Fruits
Fish
Vegetables

MAGNESIUM

It is important in resisting arteriosclerosis. It is involved in the function of the nerves and brain. There is some evidence that a deficiency can contribute to alcoholism and it is known that alcohol intake causes magnesium to be excreted in the urine. This depletion causes jumpy nerves. Adelle Davis says, in her book *Let's Get Well,* "No other single deficiency is responsible for the widespread use of tranquilizers."

Dosage. RDR—400 mg; Adelle Davis, 600-900 mg.

Must be taken with calcium for maximum use of both.

CALCIUM

Needed for good bone quality, heart function, good teeth, gums (essential for supporting dentures). Must be taken with magnesium, which controls the amount of calcium in the bloodstream. Without this control too much can get to the kidneys and lungs, causing deposits. It is especially important after menopause, when women develop a porous bone condition, causing the widow's hump and shortening of the spinal column. Take your calcium now and avoid all of this.

Dosage: RDR—1 gram (1,000 mg).

Must be taken in easily found tablets combined with magnesium.

Calcium is found in:

Milk
Cheese

IODINE

This is a necessary addition to the diet for losing weight because it helps the thyroid control the metabolism. Its absorption into the thyroid glands is greatly increased with vitamin E. Deficiencies have been known to cause goiters, high blood cholesterol, heart, and mental problems.

Dosage: RDR—150 mcg. Other nutritionists go as high as 4 mg. Since 1 mg equals 1,000 mcg, this represents a 3,850 mcg difference. Is there any wonder that there is a constant battle to get the Food and Drug Administration to raise their recommended dosage, when disparities in thinking are this great?

Iodine is found in:

Iodized salt
Kelp tablets
Sea salt

TRACE MINERALS

Copper, manganese, zinc, cobalt, and others are needed in the body in very minute amounts but a deficiency in any one can cause very large troubles.

Dosage: No RDR rating. Available in tablet form but considered adequate in a good diet.

Trace minerals are found in:

- Seafoods
- Torula yeast
- Kelp
- Green leafy vegetables

SELIUM

I am including this obscure mineral because of its relationship to our age group. It is being tested right now for us in a potential youth medication. It is extremely dangerous if overdosed, which won't be a problem to you as you would have to get a prescription for it.

Dosage: No known quantity.

Selium is found in:

- Herring
- Wheat germ
- Tuna
- Bran
- Broccoli
- Brewer's yeast
- Cabbage

SULFUR AMINO ACIDS

The "free radical" theory of aging is a popular one with biochemists and the sulphur amino acids retard their formation. A simple description of "free radicals" is that they are cells or parts of cells that are affected by pollution, radiation, and bad nutrition. They then attack healthy cells, causing further destruction.

Dosage: No RDR rating. Suggested by Dr. Kugler in his book *Slowing Down the Aging Process;* 400-600 mg, which is his daily intake—and he is a lot younger than I am.

LECITHIN

A group of compounds containing phosphorous and a fatlike substance found throughout the body. It is manufactured by the body under normal circumstances and it controls the cholesterol in the bloodstream. Therefore, it is very important to anyone facing possible arteriosclerosis. It is described as a soapylike substance, which dissolves the artery-obstructing fat particles of cholesterol. For the cook, the best way to demonstrate its action is to use it in a gravy where there is a lot of fat riding on top. Watch it absorb the fat.

Dosage: No RDR rating. The most commonly suggested amount is two tablespoons daily. I take one capsule plus this amount in a glass of milk every morning. I believe that everyone over forty should be preventing any artery trouble.

The End

For those of you who had your interest aroused by this capsule rundown of supplements, check the bibliography at the end of this chapter. I hope you have taken to heart at least one thing that will give you a more beautiful and a healthier life.

If you will allow me to reminisce about a personal experience, I have just had my yearly physical examination. This is the year I lost ten pounds, added a number of vitamins to my diet, and tried to make every food I ate a useful one. Results: cholesterol from 149 to 105; blood sugar, from 154 to 90; and, best of all, a miraculous improvement in a lung condition. This certainly proved to me that if you give those cells the right nourishment they will respond and make for better health and possibly add to your life-span.

There are eight theories being worked on right now to extend the life-span. Dr. Kugler, in his book, which I referred to earlier, claims that within the next ten years we will each take a pill every day that will add years to our lives. Beautiful! Most of these theories have their base in slowing down the deterioration of the cell, which we have the ability to control ourselves now by avoiding pollution, emotional stress, bad nutrition, excessive smoking, use of alcohol, and lack of exercise.

In the meantime, in Germany, there is a method already in use called Regenerson shots. These shots are of nucleic acid taken from embryonic animal organs. They are specifically taken from the organ of the animal and injected in the same organ of the human. They are expensive and available only in Germany. Their success has been established and accepted there.

There is another European rejuvenation process developed by Dr. Ana Aslan in Rumania. This involves the injection of procaine and has been highly publicized because of the celebrities who have gone to her for treatments. It consists of three injections a week for four weeks and must be repeated periodically for life. She also has a youth pill called H-3 or gerovital, which is available in Mexico, West Germany, Belgium, Switzerland, and England. Its results are subject to controversy. Maybe, someday?

Why have I gone to all this trouble to list the foods where these body requirements are found and the dosages for supplementing them? Take the processed foods that are either overheated or filled with preservatives, both of which destroy the vitamins. Add to this the large amounts of food required to get your daily needs in the case of some vitamins. Add to that the insecticides that have been sprayed on our grains and vegetables and deposited into the soil that grows our root vegetables. Due to their toxicity, they have destroyed some of the food value.

A friend of mine was teasing me about my tray of vitamins the other day. I said, "You only get one, you know." And it is surely true that you only get one body and only you can take care of it.

"To Your Health"

I have gathered together a list of body malfunctions and the vitamins and minerals that have been found effective to combat them. Some of these results have been shown to be successful with small groups and do not constitute scientific fact. Some of the successes are only the result of experiment with laboratory animals, which is not accepted by the American Medical Association as relating to humans. My purpose in presenting this list is to show both the proven and potential help possible from the use of vitamins and minerals.

Acne: A
Appetite: Folic acid
Arthritis: Calcium, pantothenic acid, niacinamide, E, Magnesium, B-2, C, A, B-6
Antibodies (to combat infection): C
Anemia: B-6, E, Folic Acid, B-12
Atherosclerosis: C, B-6, E, Lecithin, B-12, Inositol, choline
Arteriosclerosis: Niacinamide, Inositol, calcium, lecithin, choline
Alcoholism: B-1, Folic acid, Pantothenic acid, choline, magnesium
Aging process: B-12, lecithin, A, C, magnesium, sulphur amino acids
Alertness: Lecithin, niacinamide
Asthma: B-12
Aging skin: E, A
Allergies: Pantothenic acid, B-6, C, E

Backache: C
Bad breath: B-6
Blood pressure (high): Lecithin, choline, C
Bone strength: C, Calcium
Birth control pills: B-6
Blood vessels: C, P

Brain cells: Lecithin, niacinamide, inositol
Blood sugar (high): Pantothenic acid
Bruising: C, P, E
Burns: E, PABA, C, Pantothenic acid, calcium gluconate, B-complex
Blood clots: E, Calcium, Magnesium, linolenic acid, C
Blood coagulations: P, C, K

Common cold: C, P
Constipation: Pantothenic Acid, Lecithin, F (oils)
Cholesterol (high): Niacinamide, E, Lecithin, B-12, C
Circulation: E, Lecithin
Cortizone (if being medicated by): Potassium, Pantothenic acid, Multivitamins
Colitis: Pantothenic acid, A, E, Potassium, Magnesium, B-6, Folic acid, lecithin, niacinamide, B-complex

Digestion: B-1, B-complex, pantothenic acid, inositol, potassium
Diabetes: Inositol, B-6, magnesium, potassium, pantothenic acid, C, E
Diarrhea: B-complex, B-6, magnesium, folic acid, lecithin, niacinamide, A, B-1
Deafness: B-complex, E, iodine (kelp)

Eyes: A, B-12, B-2, Lecithin, Pantothenic acid, C, Inositol
Eczema: B-complex, F, B-6, biotin, PABA, niacinamide, magnesium, Pantothenic acid
Emphysema: E, A, C, Folic acid, Pantothenic acid

Fatigue: Pantothenic acid, Kelp, E, C
Forgetfulness: Niacinamide
Fever: B-1

Gums: Calcium, C
Gall bladder: Choline
Glaucoma: B-2

Hair: Pantothenic acid (for graying), PABA, Inositol (balding), Choline, Folic acid

Heart: E, Lecithin, Inositol, Choline, Iodine, Potassium, Magnesium
Hemorrhoids: B-6
Hay fever: A
Healing (after surgery): B-2, B-6, Copper, Magnesium, C, E, F (fatty acids), Folic acid
Headaches: B-6, Pantothenic acid, B-1, B-12

Infections: Pantothenic acid, C, Lecithin, Choline, A, B-6
Irritability: C, Lecithin, Pantothenic acid, Magnesium
Insomnia: Calcium, Magnesium, B-6, Pantothenic acid

Kidneys: A, E, Pantothenic acid, Choline, Potassium

Lungs: A, Niacinamide, C, E, Lecithin, Pantothenic acid, Folic acid
Liver: Lecithin, B-2, Pantothenic acid, Choline, C, A, E
Leg cramps: B-6, Magnesium

Muscle coordination: B-1, B-6, choline
Mucous membrane: A, B-2
Mental disorders: Niacinamide, Pantothenic acid, Inositol, Lecithin
Mononucleosis: B-6, C
Measles: A
Metabolism: B-2, Iodine
Muscle relaxers: C, Magnesium
Muscle soreness: C

Nervous exhaustion: Lecithin, Pantothenic acid
Nerves: Choline
Nephritis (kidney infection): E

Obesity: E, Pantothenic acid, B-6, Lecithin, Iodine, Potassium B-complex

Pellagra (subclinical is prevalent): Niacinamide
Pain: Calcium, K
Phlebitis: E, C
Psoriasis: Lecithin, A, B-6
"The Pill": B-6, E, Folic acid

Rhinitis (runny nose): A

Respiratory infections: Pantothenic acid

Sinus infection: A
Sore throat: B-2
Shock: C, E, B-complex
Stamina: B-complex
Sex: Lecithin, Pantothenic acid, E, Kelp, A
Scar tissue (prevents): E
Stress: Pantothenic acid, A, Linoleic acid (F), B-2, E, C
Strokes (prevention): Lecithin
Sunburn: PABA
Stretch marks: E, Pantothenic acid
Skin: B-6, A, Pantothenic acid
   Wrinkled skin: B-Complex, Lecithin
   Skin eruptions: B-2
   Some skin infections: Lecithin
   Aging skin: Lecithin, E, PABA (prescription)
   Discoloration blotches: PABA (prescription)
   Dry skin: A, C, F, B-complex
   Oily skin: B-2

Teeth: Calcium, B-6
Thyroid (hyper): Kelp, Pantothenic acid, E, Lecithin
Tranquilizers: Lecithin, C, Magnesium
Tissue repair (bruises, cuts, operations): Pantothenic acid, A, B-2, E, C, Linoleic acid (F)
Tuberculosis: C, Pantothenic acid, B-6

Ulcers: E, B-6, C, Pantothenic acid, A, D, B-complex

Varicose veins: E

Wrinkles: B-2, (for pucker lines around the mouth), B-complex, Lecithin

"Youth vitamin": Pantothenic acid

Remember that this list is not to be used on your own to cure whatever ails you. When there is a condition and not an illness, it only seems logical to me to make sure that you are getting these vitamins in some form or other; in food, separately, or in multi-vitamin capsules. It has been informative to me in guiding my choice of supplements to note the frequency of appearance of each of them. Do not let statistics fool you, however. These are some that are not in the following list of the top ten that are very important to the human needs:

C: 41
E: 38
Pantothenic acid: 30
Lecithin: 26
B-6: 24

A: 21
B-2: 14
Niacinamide: 12
Magnesium: 12
Choline: 11

Bibliography

Cantor, Alfred J. *Dr. Cantor's Longevity Diet*. New York: Award Books, 1971.
Clark, Linda. *Stay Young Longer*. New York: Pyramid Books, 1961.
Davis, Adelle. *Let's Get Well*. New York: Harcourt, Brace & World, Inc., 1965.
Dicyan, Erwin. *Vitamin E and Aging*. New York: Pyramid Books, 1972.
Ebon, Martin. *Which Vitamins Do You Need?*. New York: Bantam Books, 1974.
Gomez, Joan. *How Not to Die Young*. New York: Pocket Books, 1973.
Hauser, Gaylord. *Be Happier & Healthier*. New York: Fawcett, 1972.
———. *Mirror, Mirror on the Wall*. New York: Fawcett: Crest, 1960.
Kugler, Hans. *Slowing Down the Aging Process*. New York: Pyramid, 1974.
Lappe, Frances Moore. *Diet for a Small Planet*. New York: Ballantine Books, 1971.
McKenna, Marylou. *Revitalize Yourself*. New York: Hawthorn Books, 1972.
Pauling, Linus. *Vitamin C and the Common Cold*. San Francisco: W. H. Freeman, 1970.

Podair, Simon. *Consumer's Guide to Good Health.* New York: Pyramid Books, 1974.

Shute, Wilfred. *Vitamin E for Ailing and Healthy Hearts.* New York: Pyramid Books, 1974.

U.S. Department of Health, Education and Welfare. *F.D.A. Consumer's Memo,* 74–2010, July 1975.

Watson, George. *Nutrition and Your Mind.* New York: Harper & Row, 1972.

Williams, Roger. *Nutrition Against Disease.* New York: Pitman, 1971.

Youmans, John B. "Deficiencies of Fat Soluble Vitamins," *AMA Journal,* vol. 144, September 2, 1950.

———. "Deficiencies of Water Soluble Vitamins," *AMA Journal,* vol. 144, September 23, 1950.

6
Exercise and Stay Young

Satchel Paige, the famous old baseball player said, "Keep the juices flowing by jangling around." Isn't that a priceless description of exercising? So let us "jingle around" a little. But, before we start, let's see what our doctor has to say about it.

For those of you who have no extra weight, don't leave now. You don't exercise to lose weight but to control where you want that weight to be.

You exercise for circulation. If you are young enough to think you don't have any circulation problems, listen to this: Doctors, in examining young men for the Vietnam war found a large percentage with the start of arteriosclerosis, many with quite advanced cases. The late doctor, Dr. Irving Mendelson, said, "You start clogging your arteries at sixteen and it just doesn't catch up to you until later." Circulation carries oxygen to all parts of the body and helps to remove the toxic wastes. These wastes are what is not used by the body as a result of metabolism. One of the theories of aging has to do with toxic materials being removed more slowly as we get older. So get those juices flowing, girls!

Exercise for sagging skin. It is vital for those of you who are dieting to combine your diet with exercise. As you reduce the supporting layer of fat, the outside layer becomes looser. You need to exercise the muscles to keep that skin in place. Don't get frightened when you lose a few pounds and your skin begins to hang a little. With the good nutrition you are now aware of, exercise, and the slow weight-reduction program I have suggested, you will tighten that skin quickly.

I had two rolls of sagging fat on either side of my lower back just above the waist. If you have tried to buy a bathing suit lately you will know why those two bumps were a disaster. Those suits with deeply scooped backs were all I could find to buy. Well, one year and many exercises later, I have lost those rolls and gained a beautiful new coral suit. I am very proud.

You exercise for muscular strength. Muscles waste away from lack of use at any age but as we get older we may settle for a sedentary life too soon and accelerate the wasting. Every time I see an older person struggling to get up and down curbs, stairs, on and off buses, I wonder how much of their obvious stiffness is due to arthritis or just plain laziness—no exercise.

I was working on choreography for an amateur theatrical group about ten years ago when I tried out a step that required hopping on one foot. I couldn't do it. What a shock! My work at that time required sitting eight hours a day. I used to get in the car, drive home, and sit all evening, resting from the day's work. Sound familiar? (Footnote: I can do that step now.)

You should exercise if you have trouble with your back. I am including this because our civilization seems to be infested with back troubles. Dr. Hans Krause has written a book called simply *Backache*. He points out in his book that there is a prevalency of muscles becoming just too weak to support the body weight; this puts too much strain on the back muscles. We will get into some exercises later that are recommended by Dr. Krause, but if you have constant and severe back trouble, see your doctor. There is another group working on back problems. The theory is based on a study made by an Englishman back in the early 1900s. It is called the "Alexander Principle," and therapists now have clinics in New York, England, and Switzerland, and will bring experts to your community as well, to conduct special sessions based on it. The theory is based on posture, which starts with the proper balance of the head. When held properly, the whole body weight is carried from the neck vertebrae through the trochanter of the thighbone to slightly behind the malleolus bone of the ankle. This puts the body balance all back and up. Great for the older citizen, who is inclined to lean forward at the waist.

You exercise for mobility and agility, and this is an area I feel so strongly about that I am devoting the whole chapter following to it. If you master the art of movement, you may qualify for "Mature Beauty, U.S.A."

You exercise to relax. Physical therapists will tell you that it is just as important to relax the muscles as to stretch them. Yoga, which has become so popular as an exercise method, is a good example of this. This is a particularly good form of exercise as your stamina for strenuous exercise decreases. Your muscles stretch and relax and do not require the endurance of calisthenics or competitive sports.

You exercise for your body functions: lungs, intestines, colon, kidneys, liver, and the endocrine glands. Why? Because the stepped-up circulation carries the blood to all parts of the body faster and stimulates their action. Yoga exercises actually squeeze vital organs, massaging them to induce circulation.

What can this mean for your better health? You will have better digestion, better elimination, better breathing, so important in our air-polluted world; and for better action of our glands, so important to our body mechanism—including our sexual energy.

Doctors will tell you that there is no age limit to exercising at the right level of endurance and strain. Be sure to let your doctor tell you this, however. My eighty-six-year-old Aunt Claire has just been given a set of exercises by her doctor. I am delighted, because I have been thinking for some time that she was capable of a lot more activity than she allowed herself.

Here are my Rule of Ten exercises, divided into five parts of the body, each of which should be covered every day. These exercises should take about 10 minutes.

HEAD AND SHOULDERS

1. *Sitting.* Relax your shoulders, keeping your back straight. Drop your chin to your chest and hold for 5 counts. Raise your chin and drop your head back and hold for 5 counts. This time, take a deep breath, letting it out as you drop your chin back to your chest. Repeat 5 times each way.

2. *Sitting.* Place your hands at the back of your neck, elbows out. Now, scoop your elbows forward with a downward scoop and lift them as high as you can right up next to your ears. Add to this by taking a deep breath on each upward swoop and letting it out as you relax. Repeat 5 times.

UPPER ARMS AND CHEST

You have been aware of the unsightliness of flabby upper arms. Don't let this happen to you. If it's too late, get going!

1. *Standing.* Lock your fingers together; not interlace but lock. Got it? Raise them to bust level, elbows out, shoulders down, back straight. Pull, pull hard 10 times. Be sure that the back of one hand is facing toward you and the other away from you.

2. *Standing.* Arms straight in front at shoulder level. Swing them sharply overhead 10 times. Now, arms in the same forward position, swing them down and back as far as you can 10 times.

WAIST AND ABDOMEN

1. *On your back.* Pull your knees up with your feet on the floor. Your arms are at your sides. Lift your head from the floor as far as possible, at the same time lifting your hands to your knees. Relax.

While you are relaxing put your hand on your stomach and take a deep breath way down into your stomach making your hand rise. Push with your hand to exhale the air. You are now doing yoga breathing, very important for taking oxygen to all parts of your body. Do the exercise 10 times, taking the air in as you relax and letting it out as you reach for your knees.

2. *On your back.* Raise both feet, bringing your legs perpendicular to the floor. Kick your feet back and forth 10 times. Lower them halfway to the floor and repeat the kicks 10 times. Now, one foot from the floor, 10 times. This last is a toughie.

HIPS AND THIGHS

1. *On your back.* Arms stretched out to the side. Bend your knees to your chest. Roll from side to side, touching the floor with your knee as you reach each side. Keep your shoulders on the floor. 10 times, 5 on each side.

2. *Standing.* Tuck your bottom in by shooting your hips forward. Come up on your toes and bend your knees. This will be as though you were going to sit. Come up and take a deep breath way down into your stomach as you are going up on your toes. Bend your knees and bound 5 times exhaling for the 5 counts. Hold onto a sturdy chair if your balance is bothering you. Repeat 5 times.

LEGS AND FEET

1. *Sit in a chair.* Legs straight out ahead at chair seat level. Rotate your ankles in opposite directions. 10 times out and 10 times in.

2. *Jump on both feet 10 times.* Then from one foot to the other 10 times. How long has it been since you have jumped rope?

Do this series of exercises for one week. By the third day you will probably have them memorized. Just think of the five parts of the body and two exercises for each part and you will have it. Next week we can go on to the new set of 10 below. The following set should take about 14 minutes.

NECK AND SHOULDERS

1. *Bend at the waist, legs apart.* Clasp your hands back of you and pull up as hard as you can. Repeat 5 times.

2. *Sitting on the floor.* Twist your head as far to the right as possible. Then to the left, 5 times on each side. Now drop your head to your shoulder, keeping your shoulders pulled down. Then to the other side, each side 5 times. This area of the body needs relaxing more than any other because in this small channel all the nerves and blood vessels pass to and from the brain.

UPPER ARMS AND CHEST

1. *Standing.* Arms out to the sides at shoulder level. Make fists. Rotate your arms 10 times forward and 10 times backward. Then shake and shake and shake them.

2. *Stand two feet from a blank wall, feet apart.* Put your hands on the wall at shoulder level. Lower yourself to the wall until your nose touches. Push hard back to the original position. Do this 10 times.

WAIST AND STOMACH

1. *Standing.* Hands on hips. Bend forward as far as you can with your head looking forward. Bounce 5 times. Bounce 5 times bending to the right, 5 times to the left, and 5 times bending back. Do the whole sequence 5 times.

2. *On your back.* Arms out. Swing your left leg over and touch your right hand with your left foot. Reverse. Do this 5 times on each side.

HIPS AND THIGHS

1. *On the floor.* Turn on your right side. Raise your upper body from the floor, supporting your head with your hand, elbow on the floor. Legs together. All set? Kick your top leg to the ceiling 5 times. It pulls the leg muscles better if you flex your foot. Alternate sides, 10 counts each side.

2. *Standing*. Feet apart, arms over your head. Lunge to the right, taking all your weight on the right foot. Now bend sideward toward the left foot. Hold for 5 counts. Reverse to the left leg, 5 times on each side. One of my favorite exercises, because it uses so many muscles in legs, waist, shoulders, buttocks.

LEGS AND FEET

1. *Standing*. Deep knee bends. Hold onto the sink or washbowl. Lower yourself to the floor with your back straight. That part is easy, coming up is tougher. Keep your heels planted firmly and use your arms to pull you up at first. I give this one exercise the credit for my new ease of movement, especially stair climbing. It develops muscles in the buttocks required for lifting the body.

2. *Standing*. Feet straight ahead. Raise up on your toes 10 times. Now, bend your knees with your heels on the floor 10 times. This is the old ballet rule that if you pull the muscles in one direction, you must compensate with the opposite pull.

The above sets of exercises will give you enough variety. You can mix them up, using your own combinations but always giving yourself at least one in each area of the body. I sometimes do more in my shoulders if I am on a posture kick. You will know where your bad points are and want to work on them a little more from time to time. I can't stress enough that you should do something every day to add years and beauty to your life. And for that reason, I am going to direct the following to those of you who have just said to yourselves, "I just can't get myself to exercise."

Here is a set of exercises based on daily living:

IN BED

1. *Lift your knees with your feet planted on the mattress.* Lift your hips with your weight on your shoulders. 5 times. If your bed partner or roommate thinks you've flipped, he/she will get used to it.

2. *Lie on your right side and keeping the left leg straight.* Pull your right knee to your chest. Repeat on the left side. Do 5 times on each side.

IN BATHTUB

1. *Fill the tub until the water covers your lower back.* Reach forward and grab either your ankles or your toes. Relax and let gravity carry your head down to your knees. You won't believe how much closer you are to your knees after a slow count of 10.
2. *Fill the tub high.* Lower yourself back onto your elbows. Push the end of the tub with the ball of one foot and then the other, holding each to the count of 10. Watch what happens to your stomach when you push.

WALKING AROUND THE HOUSE

1. *Walking to the bathroom?* Lift your knee to your chest at every step. You are sure to have 10 steps. I have 15.
2. *From the kitchen to the dining room?* Raise up on your toes at every step. (Don't do this while carrying the soup.)

WAITING IN LINE AT THE SUPERMARKET

1. *Pull your buttocks together—hard.* Hold for 10 counts. What happens to your stomach? The muscles pull in and up and it flattens right out. The fun is that no one can see you doing this, so you can do it anytime you think about it. At least, I hope you are not wearing slacks that are too tight.
2. *Stretch your head up, up, up, wherever you are, but the supermarket line is such a bore, it will give you something to think about.*

IN THE SHOWER

1. *A great time to stretch your neck and exercise it against the coming sag.* Jut your chin forward and tip your head back. Now,

move your jaw from side to side. Try this with the water splashing in your face. Wow! This will ward off that double chin. Do 20 times.

2. *Hands on your shoulders, elbows out.* Twist your waist from side to side as far around as you can get. Don't let your hips turn. Do 10 times on each side.

AT THE BREAKFAST TABLE

1. *While you are chewing your first mouthful, put your spoon down, grasp the edge of the table with both hands and push your back hard against the back of the chair. Stretch!* Doesn't that feel great? Do for 10 counts.

2. *Hands under the seat of the chair on each side, straighten your arms and pull up. Hold for 10 counts.*

WATCHING TV

1. Even though Clarence has just told Gertrude that he loves another woman and the telephone is ringing to tell them that their daughter has just been hit by a truck, you can still take your shoes off and press hard against the floor with the balls of your feet. If you are not too glued, try to notice that you are using your leg muscles, thigh and foot muscles, to say nothing of your stomach.

2. *Everyone else is watching the tube so you can try a facial exercise without being caught.* So, clench your teeth and open one side of your mouth with the other remaining closed. Lifts the whole side of your face, doesn't it? Relax the muscles slowly and repeat on the other side. Do 5 times on each side.

PICKING UP

1. *Drop this book on the floor!* Pick it up. Did you bend your back or your knees? I hope it was your knees and if not, here is the way to save your back. Put one foot about six inches in back of the other, foot flexed so the weight is on the ball of that foot. Swoop

down with your knees bent and *voila!* It won't be cheating to push off from the floor with your free hand.

2. *Pick up that chair.* Did you lean over, using only the muscles of your back? Try it again, turning your feet parallel to the chair with the foot closest to the chair behind the other and flexed, weight on the ball again. Bend your knees, lift, and you have done it all with your legs. Eric Taylor, author of *Stay Young Forever,* a noted authority on physical fitness, preaches against the common practice of using your back instead of your legs. He wants you to bend your knees rather than your back every time you reach for your shoes in the closet or get something from the bottom shelf of the refrigerator. Save your back.

TALKING ON THE PHONE

1. *If you talk on the phone as much as I do, you can get your whole day's exercises done right there.* It is true that you can set up a stimulous–response situation at the phone or in any other daily circumstance that triggers a given exercise. Try this one for the phone. Come up on your toes and bend your knees as though you were going to sit. Keep your back straight and your fanny tucked in. Bounce 5 times. This is a repeat from the Hip and Thigh exercises and a very important one.

2. *Stretch the arm that is not holding the phone over your head.* Bend to the side, bounding 5 times. Change the phone and bend the other way. I hope Virginia, on the other end, doesn't notice a shortness of breath.

Whatever approach you take, exercise will make you feel younger and look younger. Doctors encourage them at any age if they are geared to your physical capacity. Check with your doctor to find any limitations he may want to place, and follow his advice. Keep jangling so those juices will flow.

Bibliography

Allean, Robert. *The Art of Staying Younger*. New York: Simon & Schuster, Franklin Essaudes Special Editions, 1964.
Barton, Wilfred. *The Alexander Principle*. London: Victor Gollancz, Ltd., 1973.
Beck, Toni, and Swank, Patsy. *Fashion Your Figure*. Boston: Houghton Mifflin, 1973.
Ford, Eileen. *A More Beautiful You in 21 Days*. New York: Simon & Schuster, 1972.
Krause, Hans. *Backache*. New York: Simon & Schuster, 1965.
McKenna, Mary Lou. *Revitalize Yourself*. New York: Hawthorn Books, 1972.
Taylor, Erik. *Stay Young Forever*. New York: Arco, 1972.
Walker, Morton. *Your Guide to Foot Health*. New York: Arco, 1972.

7
Move Like a Teen-ager in 10 Easy Lessons

Uncle Joseph was as straight as a ramrod until the day he died. Did you have one of those in your family? He was certainly admired by all, but a terrible burden to a growing child. "Why can't you stand up straight like your uncle?" I sure wish I had now.

Bad posture can be a problem at any age, but the stoop of anyone in an older group is accepted as part of the aging process. I don't agree. Muscle action can be explained this way: The flexor muscles go with gravity and demand very little effort. The extensor muscles must be pulled against gravity and take a lot more effort. Through the years of making less and less effort, you can end up with a sunken chest and a rounded back if you don't start now to avoid it. This can be true of your shoulders. It is easy to let them fall forward more and more. How about your knees? Do you keep them perpetually bent?

Well, isn't it great to know that these unused muscles can be rejuvenated? If you want to take ten years off of your looks get your posture straightened out. Get over to that full-length mirror we spoke of earlier. You are facing directly into it. You can't see the slouch that way! Maybe the slouch has developed because you have been looking at yourself from this direction right along. Turn sideways. If you are lucky, all those nasty things I said in the last paragraph won't apply to you. If you are lucky you will be a straight line from the tip of your spine to the base of your neck. Not so straight? Pull in your stomach and push out your chest. What has happened to your fanny? If it is sticking out, causing a curve in your back, shoot your hips forward like the burlesque queen's "bumps." When you have all of that, lean your whole torso back a little so that your weight will follow down the back leg muscles to your heels.

Rule of Ten for better posture:

1. Walk over to the closest wall and line your back up against it. Put your hand between the wall and the small of your back. If there is a wide open space there, there shouldn't be. Contract the muscles in your buttocks and your back straightens up. Push hard with the ball of your left foot and your backbone is solid against the wall from top to bottom. Push 10 times with each foot.

2. Lie on your back with your arms at your sides. Press your elbows hard against the floor. Now push hard with your head, then your heels. Hold for 5 counts and repeat 5 times.

3. Standing. Stretch your arms over your head, shoulders down. Shoot one arm higher and stretch it. Alternate arms and count to 20, 10 with each arm. Keep your hips forward!

4. Lie on your stomach with your arms stretched out in front. Lift your head. Then lift your arms alternately as far as they will go, giving your back a good stretch. Do 5 times with each arm. Good for your back, too.

5. Stay in this position. Lift your head back as far as you can and hold it for 5 counts. Do 5 times. Try it with a heavy book on the back of your neck.

6. Standing. Bend your elbows. Pull your left elbow back, keeping the right shoulder straight ahead. Do 5 times on each side.

7. Standing. Both arms over your head, shoulders down. Pull back hard 10 times. Spread arms apart about 4 feet. Repeat. Lower arms to shoulder level and repeat 10 times.

8. Walk across the floor, stretching the top of your head to the ceiling. Carrying on it the proverbial book, perhaps. It may sound corny, but it works, and it's fun.

9. Get down on your knees and sit back on your heels. Now fall forward on your hands. Lower your chin to the floor. Repeat 5 times. Mini push-ups, and great for the shoulders and chest muscles.

10. Back to the mirror. Pull your head up, stick your chest out, pull your stomach in, shoot your hips forward, pull the whole torso back. Hold 10 counts. Relax. Repeat 5 times.

I am aware that this is all too much to think of at the same time. So let us take them one at a time. Today, think ten times, wherever you are or whatever you are doing: "Pull your stomach in." Tomorrow say to yourself ten times: "Stretch your head up to the ceiling." Each day take another correction, one at a time: shoulders back, chest up, hips tucked forward, lean the torso back. Then take a day to put them all together ten times. I have to keep working constantly at my posture, so I vary this to maybe a whole week of remembering to lift my head to the ceiling ten times a day. I heard an important sociologist say on television recently that her biggest hope for the future of mankind was increased self-awareness. This can be your salvation. By saying: "Pull your stomach in" ten times a day you aren't just drifting.

YOUNG MOVEMENT TAKES OFF YEARS

One of the first things a model learns is to "lead with the shoulder." This action turns the waist and shows off the clothes better. Try it. Stand with your hands on your hips. How far can you turn your torso without moving your hips? Now let one shoulder pull as far forward as you can. If you can't move very much your back muscles are stiff. This won't do if you are going to move like a ballerina.

Rule of Ten to rejuvenate muscles and regain younger movements:

1. Stand sideways to your closet and reach across your body for a hanger, keeping your hips from moving.

2. Walk 5 steps forward and turn. Did you shuffle your feet, changing your weight several times before getting around? Try it again: 1, 2, 3, 4, 5, on the ball of your foot and swivel. All your weight is on this foot, you are turned, and you have a foot free on which to step out in the opposite direction. This is the model pivot. Get this one and you will be a model yet. That isn't so funny. Many stores use matron models in their style shows.

3. When you get the pivot on the ball of your foot, try this. Open a door slightly, so your body will only go through sideways. Go through the opening your way. Ten to one you sidestepped your way through. Try it with your weight on the ball of your foot. Swivel, swing the opposite shoulder through the opening and in one movement you are ready to step out again on the other side.

4. Let's sit down. Most women give no thought to this daily movement, which classifies them as a frump at any age if they clump into a chair, usually with their knees spread. Here's how: Approach the chair sideways so that when you lower yourself your knees will stay together. Just as you get to the chair take your weight on the balls of your feet and swivel. Neat, and all without bending at the waist, I hope.

5. Getting up? First try this in a chair with a shallow seat. Turn both feet in the same direction so they are not directly forward. Put one foot back of the other. It has to be the one away from the chair. Push with the ball of that foot, your weight is on the front foot and, voila, you are up without any movement in the waist. If you are in a deep chair, move forward to the edge and you get the same results. If you forget this one you will soon be reminded when you watch others struggling in and out of their chairs. You will develop a pride in doing it right.

6. Now that you are sitting, look back over your shoulder. Pull your shoulder way around and keep your back straight. Remember this the next time you want to wave to Mable in the back row.

7. Having trouble getting down on the floor? It's easy. Cross your left foot way across in front of you, taking all your weight on it. Slip your right leg under you, knee bent, and drop to the floor, catching your weight with both hands crossed over to the right. This eases you down on your fanny without a thud.

8. Come up the same way. Hands on the floor, plant your left foot across in front and push with hands and foot. You are up with a minimum of effort.

9. If you ride a bus, as we all do, step up the big step without bending at the waist. This takes some doing at first. If your exercises from the previous chapter are going to pay off it will be now. The muscles in your lower leg and fanny must give you the strength to lift your body weight. When I accomplished this, I felt ten years younger.

10. Stand up. Look at your feet. Some women stand so that their feet almost form a V. This turns the knees out and inclines them to bend a little. You'll never be a model that way. If you want a more graceful standing position, turn your feet forward and bend one knee a little. This keeps the knees from turning out, it moves one hip out and the whole result is that your dress doesn't hang like a sack but has some movement to it.

Walking

My pet peeve.

Someone said, "Walk as though you were going somewhere, not already been." I think it was me.

We have already worked on our posture so that our weight is distributed straight down the backbone to the heels with the weight on the whole foot. Because we have been walking all our lives on heels that throws our weight on the ball of the foot, the muscles in the back of the leg have to be developed. Recognition of this theory has been demonstrated by college students lately: They are wearing "earth shoes," both boys and girls. The heel is actually lower than the front part of the shoe, throwing the weight completely on the heel. This exaggeration would seem to me to produce a stiff-kneed walk. Before we go into how to make you a gliding swan, let us take a look at some of the poor walking habits prevalent on our streets:

1. *"The pigeon-toed."* This condition stops the full stride, causes the knees to bend too much, and pulls the torso forward.

2. *"The wandering foot."* Those who throw their feet to the side with a little extra movement instead of stepping straight ahead. This throws the stride off and makes it jerky.

3. *"The bounder."* These people get too much action in the arch of their feet and waste too much energy going up and down—and they look funny doing it.

4. *"The slumper."* There are legitimate arthritic conditions that cause a forward lean. If that is not your trouble, stand up, pull your shoulders back, and lean back a little. Don't slouch for the life of you. This is not only a telltale sign of age, but it indicates a negative attitude toward the world.

5. *"The duck foot."* This is putting the feet down with toes turned out and wide apart, making a waddle. This is frequently caused by obesity, due to the accumulation of fat on the inner leg. This won't be you after you have had a go at your diet.

6. *"The stiff-kneed."* This produces a short, shuffly step.

7. *"The shuffler."* Advanced years bring on this condition for various reasons, one of them being decreased circulation, leaving the feet somewhat numb. So, for security, they are not lifted very far off the ground. We won't get into this situation with our leg exercises and our vitamins to keep our circulation going, will we?

8. *"The clumper."* These walkers lift their knees high and land on their foot with a clump that jerks the whole body and impedes a smooth stride.

9. *"The weak arch."* The foot rolls over onto the arch, stopping the forward movement.

Watch the walk of the people in your family and others. Try to classify them. Where do you fit?

Walking habits are developed so early in life that changing them requires a lot of work, but it's worth it. I have taken a whole year and done a lot of walking to accomplish a permanent change. Well, nearly permanent. I catch myself slouching in the waist occasionally. The thing to keep in mind when learning a new walk is *time*. Take each new thought and try to work on it until you have the correction made. When you are making a posture change with the Rule of Ten, it is just as easy to add a walking one.

Here are four ways to correct some of the problems that cause ugly walking:

1. *Pull your torso back so that your weight is on your heels as well as the ball of your foot.* Walk around the room. This pulls the muscles in the front of the thigh and down the back of your legs. They may be sore for a few days after you get into doing this 10 times a day. If they hurt, you are doing it right. Perhaps I should explain that the whole upper part of your body should be pulled up and back, not just your waist. Put your hands on your fanny and you will feel the muscles contract as you pull back. You will know how far back to lean because your balance will tell you. Keep at this one for a whole week without trying any of the other corrections.

2. *Next week try walking with your feet following a straight line in front of you.* To do this your knees have to brush slightly as they pass. This will cause a slight movement from side to side of your hips. This is no hula, but this give in the hip joint cushions the jolt when your heel hits. This must all be done with the knees slightly bent. Try it, it's fun.

3. *Let your arms swing naturally with your stride.* This should require no special attention but can be a problem if you stiffen up.

4. *The correct way to take weight on your foot is from the heel*

along the outside edge. This takes the weight forward to the toes, which grip and send you forward onto the other foot. Try this first sitting down with no weight on your foot. Heel, around the outside and onto your toes. This takes a long time to change to if you are inclined to drop the weight to the inner arch as I was. You might want to exercise your feet by curling your toes under when you think about it. I even do it in bed. Take a week to try this out: 10 times a day walk 10 steps with "heel, around, toes" on your mind.

Walking and posture go hand in hand. If you lick some of the problems of one you have automatically licked the other. You need to be beautiful in your walk for several reasons:

1. You show your clothes to a better advantage. There is no use spending money on that new Donald Brooks just to go slumping around in it.
2. A confident walk shows a confident you. Your walk reveals a great deal about you. If you watch others on the street, you will see what their walk tells you about them.
3. You are exercising the right muscles for strength in your legs. This becomes pretty important as you get older.
4. Your walk is one of the most revealing characteristics of age. Granted that there are thirty-year-olds who shuffle along as though they were eighty. You reverse it. You can learn to step out there as though you were thirty.

Want to try the stairs now? The distance between floors is much farther than it used to be, isn't it? Part of the trouble is circulation and some wasted leg muscles. With your exercises you are going to notice a lot of improvement in both. The feet should be placed on each step with the body erect. Moving from step to step involves the muscles in the buttocks as well as the leg muscles. You are working with both of these with your new walking and your deep knee bends. The most common ugliness is to bob at the waist. To lick this, bend your knees, keep your back straight, and let the muscles in your feet, lower legs, front thighs, buttocks, and back lift you. I find it easier to keep both feet aimed slightly sideways to the stairs.

Going down? Same thing, bend your knees. But this time let your ankles and feet do the work. Turn both feet angled in the same direction and you will glide down the stairs like a sixty-dollar-an-hour model.

Getting into a car can be most ungraceful at any age. At our age it is more important than ever to do it right. Turn yourself so that you are facing out from the car door. Sit, bring one foot in and then the other and you have avoided a lot of unnecessary shuffling.

Watching others is sometimes the best of lessons. Here are some of the things I have noticed that have told of fleeting youth:

1. *Riding on a bus is a wonderful way to observe humanity.* In this case, women. One morning I counted six older women lined up across from me like pigeons on a roof. There were six in various stages of collapse and slump. But number five—there she sat with her head up, her shoulders back, ready for anything, looking like a queen.

2. *Watch the mouths that are drooping around you.* You will recognize meanness, sadness, disgust, disillusionment. They all show in the mouth. When you become aware of the muscles that control these expressions, you will be able to correct them. Keep up your corners!

You will begin to notice in others many more examples that reveal age, and you will learn to avoid them. Keep remembering those flexor and extensor muscles, and don't let gravity win.

8
Wear Becoming and Fashionable Clothes

I called Norman Johnson of Saks Fifth Avenue one day to ask for an interview. I said I would like his ideas on dress for the older woman. He said, "Mrs. Seiffert, I will be glad to talk to you, but before you come I want you to know I don't believe there is such a thing. Fashion is for the individual and not for an age group." That was a beautiful thing to hear, and in the hour that this fine man talked to me, we never again referred to age. This man, who buys couturier clothes for the thirty Saks Fifth Avenue stores, also talked about comfort, which he feels to be very important in selecting a garment. He talked about body proportion rather than height as the basis for choosing length and shape of jacket and skirt. He talked about materials and colors that are best for different body structures. He talked about fashion for the individual. And that is what fashion should be all about . . . adjusting the fashion trends to you.

How to arrive at fashion? How can we keep fashion as a part of our lives without being its slave or ignoring new trends altogether? First, let us consider the fashion magazines, which are so advanced in their editorial copy and pictures that we cannot relate to them. These have a purpose. They prepare you for changes. The designer creations you are seeing now in all their extreme styling will be watered down some time later for you and me, and we will be ready for the change.

Development of fashion through the ages has been influenced by the economy, war or peace, weather, new material developments, and even inventions. How could women continue to get into the automobile with those voluminous skirts? Need for adornment showed up as early as the cavemen's drawings, where their bodies were covered with decorative paintings. Psychologically based reasons for man's choice of covering his body have become more sophisticated, but sexual attraction, from the example of animals to those of birds, is the most primitive. The female in our civilization does the attracting—although today men are coming pretty close with their color revolution. The female, throughout the history of our own Western culture has created contradictions in sexual attractions, such as the nearly bared bosom combined with the modestly hidden leg. The flapper dress of the twenties revealed the leg and lost the bosom. The recent miniskirt was also accompanied by a modest top in most cases. The modestly cut top is still with us, but when it is worn with no bras beneath the fitted knit T-shirt, it certainly ceases to be modest. What is perfectly acceptable in one generation is indecent in another.

When you buy a new coat, you reflect your psychological needs, your self-image, your social situation and, as if that weren't enough, you put on top of that your body type, your complexion, and your awareness of current fashion. You did not realize it was so complicated, did you?

The need for possessions influences what you buy. The manager of season ticket sales for a large Midwest theater told me of a customer who complained about his assigned seats for the coming season. "I didn't pay $10,000 for my wife's sable coat to sit in the eighteenth row," he explained. "I want third row center or nothing." We all have a little of this in us, you know. Don't you want everyone to see your new fall suit and admire it? I do.

Social acceptance ranks high in our clothes selection. It can be conservative or haute couture, but it should conform to the social situation that dictates your life-style. Luckily, within whatever realm, there is enough variety of choice to keep us all from looking like penguins. Remember the penguin, however, when you are making your next clothing purchase. Does your best friend have one just like it in another color? I occasionally see these "twinsies," as I call them, arm in arm, strolling down Fifth Avenue. I saw *three* together once, with the same length coat, same fur, and the same fur hat. This tendency seems prevalent in the over-fifty set, so watch out.

Our self-image has a great influence on us in picking out our clothes. You can see all around you perfect examples of this. You have a quiet friend who wears soft, inoffensive colors, a modest style, and small patterns so as not to be seen, not to be in the limelight. I am sure you can bring to mind a flamboyant friend who adores the brighest colors and the biggest patterns, made up in the most exaggerated styling. Remember "fashion is for the individual." All you have to watch out for is that you don't fall into the "Johnny's grandmother" image of yourself. That does not say that you cannot err on the other side and try to identify in the wrong age bracket. There are very few rules anymore, so you have to guess a little, but please, no blue jeans at the dinner party. Leave this craziness to the younger set.

Teach yourself to look at certain details of the garment you are buying. I was fortunate enough to have an education in construction in my somewhat later years. I got involved with a group of young designers and ultimately started a small shop with their creations. Believe me, I learned a lot and even got into some designing myself. It was the most fun I ever had in business. Here is a list of details to notice the next time you are in a fitting room, which will help you make your decision:

1. The Neckline. The flat collar has been replaced in the fashion market by one that rides much higher on the back of the neck. Remember that little flat-collared suit? This change is a problem for the shorter neck and, as in all fashion, you must look for a variation that works better for you.

The turtleneck and the cowl neckline are a godsend to the aging neck and can be found from sweaters to formals. In fact, after certain years, the décolletage of the formal blouse or gown should be watched very carefully. If you are revealing deep lines at the cleavage, don't wear the gown any more. I remember sitting next to a friend at a formal dinner and suddenly becoming aware of her age in her beautiful blue-beaded, deep-cut dress.

If the boat neck, the scoop neck, and the V-neck are becoming necklines for you, your problems are not easy. Designers may have ruled all three out for the season, and you can comb the town and find nothing but shirt collars. It is a problem.

2. The Shoulders. The natural shoulder, with either the raglan sleeve or the set-in sleeve, has been used by the designers for a long time now. With the drop of hemlines and the skirt filling out, do you suppose we are in for the heavily padded shoulders of the late forty's? The big-shouldered woman wears a raglan sleeve well, since there is no seam to draw the eye to the shoulder. The small shoulder span can be expanded by yolks both front and back or either one.

3. The Waistline. Changes in the waistline can be most ruinous to last year's garment, since they are so subtle. They can pinch in slightly this year and a little more the year after—and in a different place. The box jacket with no waist at all goes in and out of fashion, but with changes nevertheless. It can hang perfectly straight or flare slightly at the sides—or at the back. The fullness can hang from the shoulder or from the armholes.

There is the Empire waist, way up under the bust. There is the trapeze dress, with the fullness hanging from the shoulder or at bust level. There is the shift dress with no waistline at all. There is a waistline for you, and don't get carried away with the wrong one just because you like the color of the dress.

4. Sleeve Treatment. A friend and I were berating the fashion manufacturers recently for their slavish following of fashion in sleeve treatment. If cuffed sleeves are in, try to find one with loose sleeves.

Now all sleeves are not good for all figures. The short, hippy woman should not wear full or big-cuffed sleeves, which extend her girth and cut her height in two. What if that is all they are showing this season? The sleeveless or capped sleeve is for the young, and I mention these because they are on their way back. I hope they will not be the only choice we have, as they were the last time they dominated the scene. My arms are not up to it. I don't know about yours, but don't fool yourself. Take a good look.

The long, slim sleeve is most becoming, but make sure that the material does not cling to your upper arm if you have let it get too heavy. If you are tall and slim, with long arms, you can wear the full sleeve and the big cuff—and should.

The three-quarter, loose sleeve has dated a garment for some time now, but it is back in a fuller version and I, for one, rejoice. I feel liberated, dramatic, and feminine. Those tight-cuffed sleeves of the shirt blouse stifle personality, and they are hot. If you feel neater and happier in the cuffed sleeve, they are still around.

5. Skirt Length. The last few years have been unusual in the fashion world. The choice of lengths has been so wide that you can see the miniskirt and the full-length dress sitting next to each other on the subway, along with every conceivable length in between. But slowly, with the advent of the fuller skirt, hemlines are edging down. Last year's good suit may have a last year's look if you don't consider the possibilities of dropping the hem.

Not only streetwear, but your formal gowns must be watched carefully for change. Sweep the floor if you must, or shorten to the ankle bone, but don't go to that dance with last year's length if you don't want those with a fashion eye to know you are in a three-year-old number.

Cheat. Taking into account your height, you can cheat short or longer and still stay within the realm of fashion requirements. If you are tall, you cheat shorter. If you are short, you cheat longer. It's all proportion, remember.

6. Skirt Shape. Remember back to all the skirt shapes you have lived through! But, since fashion dictates are so subtle, don't think you can drag your ten-year-old number out and get by with it. The shape will be wrong, I'll bet. The term *silhouette* is just that. It is the shape of the garment as seen in solid black against a white background. Studying details will teach you to see that the old one hugs the hips too far down, flares too low, or whatever.

The straight skirt, even, can have changes. Remember the tapered skirt that curved in at the knee and hobbled you a little? A friend of mine confessed that she had to remove her dress completely when she went to the ladies' room. Mine weren't quite that tight, I guess.

The A-line skirt has been popular for some time now, and rightly so. It is comfortable and flattering to women of almost any height. The variation that has to be watched is where the flare starts. If it flares right from the hips, it is better for a taller figure than a shorter one.

Beware of the full skirt, unless you are tall and willowy with a 22-inch waist.

The pleated skirt has alway been a favorite, with pleats varying in size and placement in the skirt ad infinitum. Pleats in front and back are good for the hippy woman. Pleats at the four corners of the skirt give the skirt movement and a flare, without adding girth. Pleats sewed down to below the hips make the skirt flip nicely when you walk. If you pick the pleat that is right for you, they are young and fun.

Before we leave the skirt, there is something more to look for. If the material is right and is cut on the bias or in panels, it will move gracefully when you walk. It is feminine and sexy and gives you a feeling of drama when that material swishes around your legs. My young designers taught me this.

As you have probably observed, slacks change, too. The straight, skinny leg has blossomed out. It flares at the bottom some years—and last year's flare is not this year's flare. The straight leg that hangs from the biggest part of your buttocks is the one to look for. If it cups in and hugs the leg to the knee, forget it. Look very carefully at yourself in the rear when you are buying slacks. I wish more women would. The sights one sees! Note the change in lengths also.

Watching for these changes in details is what fashion awareness is all about. You will save yourself money by knowing that shorter skirts, big lapels, dropped waistlines are on their way in or out. You will buy clothes that are not at the end of a fashion trend and can be worn longer. Maybe you can be like a Dickens character, Mr. Boffin, whose wife was "a regular high flyer at fashion."

COLOR

I ought to announce right now that I believe color to be one of the most important features in clothes selection. You can have every detail of a garment fashion-perfect and miss the color that is good for you—and you have wasted your money. Many people who see you daily do not know or care about what is stylish, but when you are wearing a color that sparks you they say to themselves, "Doesn't Mrs. Glutz look nice today."

You are not going to enroll in an art school to learn the nuances of color so that you can select the right one every time. All of us have to rely on a "by-guess-and-by-golly" and, heaven forbid, the salesgirl.

Rule of Ten: Setting down any rules on color selection is very touchy, but these may make you stop and think:

1. Colors are more than red, white, and blue. It is in the selection of *shades* that you will find one you can wear. Shades can be too yellow or too blue for your coloring. Don't say, "I can't wear green." Maybe Kelly green is too yellow for you. Try one with more blue in it and you may be surprised. Reds vary in every direction. Blues are worse.

2. Watch the vibrancy of the color. The dictionary defines the word as "pulsing or throbbing with energy or activity." If we translate that meaning to color, we have one with some authority, one that speaks to you, even though it is beige-gray or brown. You can buy a dead-looking beige with a lot of black in it and, granted, it won't get dirty so fast, but I'll take the color that lifts the spirit every time—and pay the cleaning bills.

3. Get out of that groove. Maybe you chose a color that best suited you long ago. From your first prom dress on, this is your color. You reach for the blue suit every time and, as you have added years, the shade has become more muted. Combine this monotonous color selection with your same short-sleeved dress and the hip-length jacket and you aren't buying a dress, you are buying a uniform.

4. Don't get carried away by the styling itself, oblivious of how the color looks on you. I did this recently. Every time I put the dress on, I look in the mirror and I take it off. It ages me ten years.

5. Stay away from too-light colors at the top if you are big-busted.

6. Don't wear white pants or skirts that are too fitted if you are big in the hips.

7. Big in the waist? Break your colors from top to bottom. Light blouse, dark skirt or pants—or the reverse.

8. Keep in mind that a lighter color at the neck is always a pickup. Whistler's mother knew what she was doing with that lace collar. Today we have all kinds of choices. We have the turtleneck insert, the all-important scarf and lighter sweater, or blouses worn under darker sweaters, or a blouse with the lighter color nearest the face: the layered look.

9. Watch your color selection when you start getting gray. The salt-and-pepper stage needs solid colors. I saw a woman the other day with her salt-and-pepper tweed suit, her salt-and-pepper hat to match, and her salt-and-pepper hair wisping out under the hat, and she looked like a bolt of material walking down the street. I personally dislike some shades of brown with graying hair, but if the complexion is right for the shade, it can be effective. Redheads enlarge their color choices when gray starts to soften their hair. Some bright reds and pinks are theirs to wear, at last.

10. Complexion is the basic consideration in choosing the color you wear. You have long since known your skin tone. Maybe, however, your delicate cameo skin has sallowed up a little. Maybe you can't get by with the same shades of light pastels any more.

Black skin is the least subject to change and enviable, because every color in the spectrum enhances the black skin. The strong contrasts and the monochromatic are equally admirable.

In general, brighter colors or more vibrant tones will be better for almost any complexion when the skin gets older. There is no color that can't be worn by any age these days, so go to it. We've come a long way from grandmother's day.

SELECTING CLOTHES FOR YOUR FIGURE

Which one of these is you?

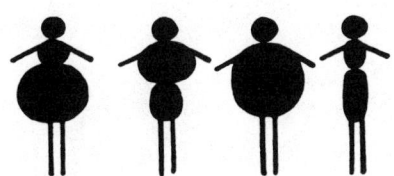

You can certainly find yourself in one of these five—with mild variations:

1. Big bottom, small bosom.
2. Big bosom, small hips.
3. No bosom, no hips.
4. Big bosom, big hips, big waist.
5. Here is where we all want to be: 34"-24"-34".

They say, aside from twins, that there are no facial structures exactly alike. I believe that the female figure must be almost as varied. Here are some do's and don'ts to help you select the right garment to hide any figure flaws.

Big Hip Do's

Flared skirts
A-line skirts
Dark skirts
Vertical designs
Big pleats sewn down below the
 biggest part of the hip
Medium to light-weight fabrics
Jackets below the largest
 part of the hip
Slacks that hang from the
 biggest part of the buttocks

Big Hip Don'ts

Clinging fabrics
Shiny fabrics
Light colors, or white in pants
 or tight skirts
Extremely short skirts
Small pleats that hang from the
 waist
Short peplums
Big prints
Horizontal stripes
Jackets fitted over the hips
Slacks that cup in at the buttocks

Small Hip Do's

Full skirts from waist
 (gathers and pleats)
Horizontal stripes
Bordered patterns
Big plaids (not too big if
 you are short)
Big patterns
Shiny materials
Heavy materials
A-line starting from waist
Straight skirts

Small Hip Don'ts

Clinging material
Slacks that cup in
Slacks with contour waistbands

Big Hip Do's

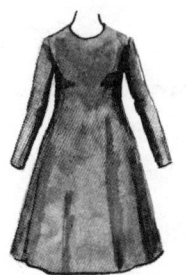
A-line

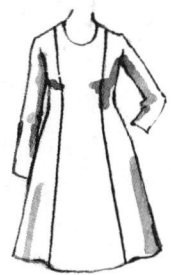
vertical seams

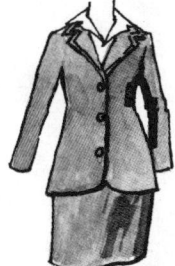
long jacket

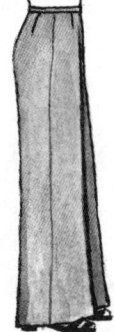
pants that hang from the buttocks

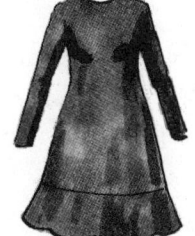
added flare or ruffled at bottom

Big Hip Don'ts

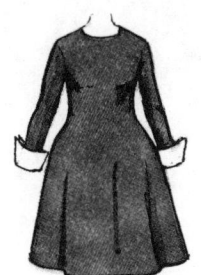
big cuffs

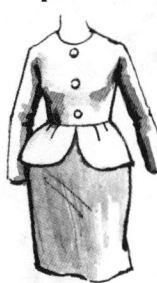
peplums

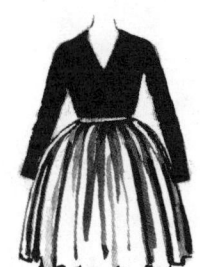
full skirts

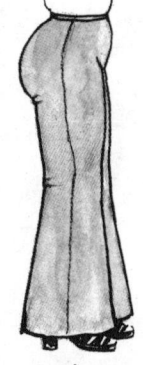
pants that cup in rear

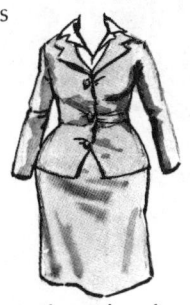
jackets that fit tightly over hips

Small Bosom Do's

Empire dresses
Trapeze dresses
Loose tops
Draped necklines
Gathers, pleats, ruffles
Big lapels
Boleros and vests
Double-breasted suits and coats
Pockets at bustline

Small Bosom Don'ts

Tight blouses, unless relieved by bow or scarf
Deep-cut necklines

Small Bosom Do's

Empire

ruffles

big lapels

pockets

Double-breasted, full lapels, buttons

Big Bosom Do's

V necklines
Small lapels
Light-weight fabrics
Dresses and blouses that button down the front
Draped and deep-cut necklines
Bust darts that start in the low part of the side seam and angle up
Vertical lines, like small tucks and seams

Big Bosom Don'ts

Clinging fabrics
Big prints
Tight blouses
Pockets at bustline
Pleats or fullness from shoulder seams
Horizontal stripes
Double-breasted suits or coats

Big Bosom Do's

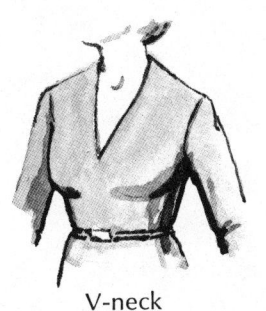
V-neck

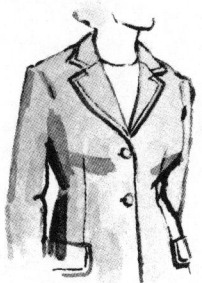
small lapels

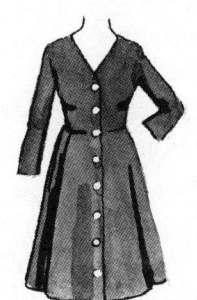
buttons down front

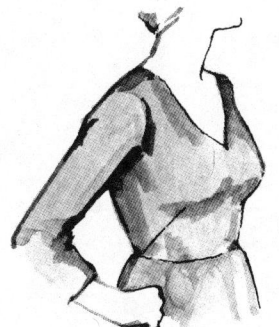
angle of dart

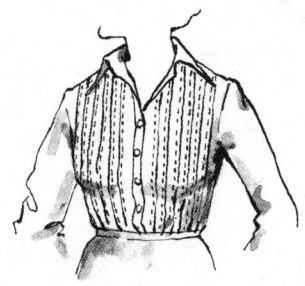
vertical tucks

Tall Thin with No Hip, No Bosom Do's

Clinging materials
A-line dresses and skirts
Full skirts from waist
Quilted cotton skirts
Heavy tweeds
Peplums
Tunics
As short a skirt as you can cheat out and still be close to the fashion
Horizontal stripes
Big armholes
Big cuffs
Big lapels
Big, full coats
Big patch pockets
Shoulder yokes
Long overblouses

Tall Thin with No Hip, No Bosom Don'ts

Tight-fitting tops and skirts together
Unbelted sheaths
Empire waistlines

Do you see, now, why the average height for a model is 5'7" and her measurements are 34"-24"-34"? There is not much they cannot wear.

Tall Do's

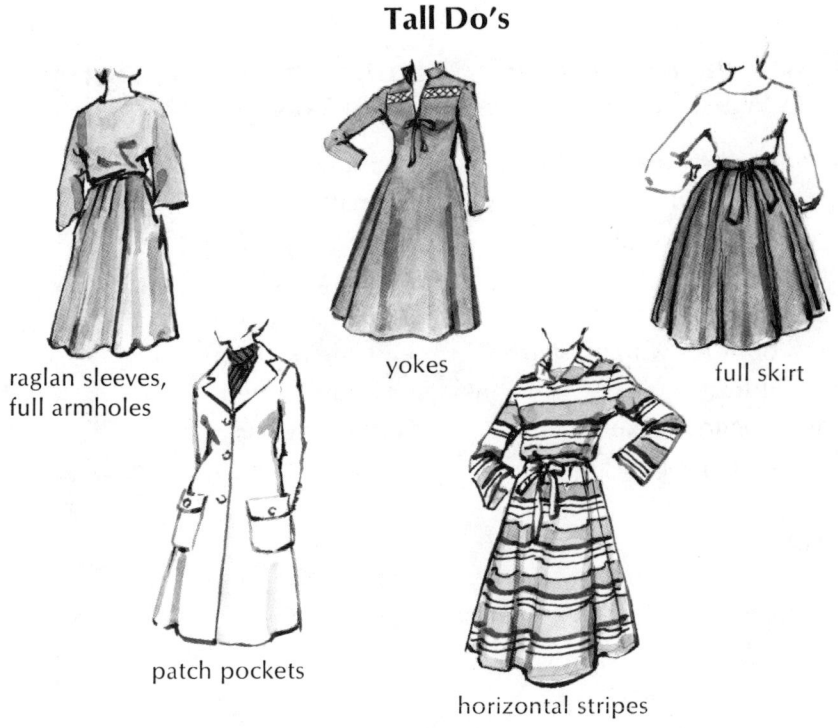

raglan sleeves, full armholes

yokes

full skirt

patch pockets

horizontal stripes

Tall Don'ts

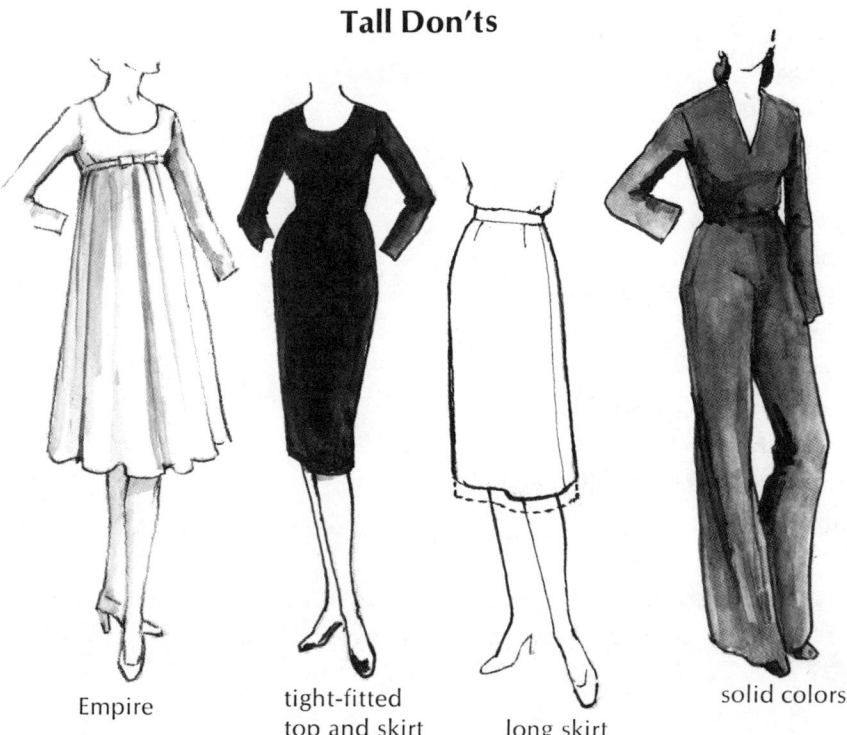

Empire

tight-fitted top and skirt

long skirt

solid colors

Short, with Big Bust, Big Hip, No Waistline Do's

Skirts and slacks with very thin or no waistbands
Slacks that hang from the buttocks
Solid colors, not too light
Tops and bottoms with no sharp color contrasts
Straight, unbelted jackets, falling below the largest part of the hip
Small lapels
Single-breasted
Vertical seams on jackets, blouses, skirts, coats
Soft materials that move
Slim arms with no cuff
Length as long as possible within the fashion dictates
A-line skirt
Straight skirt
Long overblouse
Tunics
Trapeze dresses
Draped bodices
Dresses that button down the front
V-necklines
Necklaces not beyond fullest part of bosom
Draped necklines, like the cowl
Small handbags

Short, with Big Bust, Big Hip, No Waistline Don'ts

Peplums
Big patterns
Wide belts
Shiny fabrics
Tight-fitting skirts
Outside pockets
Contrasting belts
Shoulder yokes
Big cuffs

Lucky you, if you are the perfect horizontal figure! You have only the restrictions of vertical proportion to worry about.

Short Do's

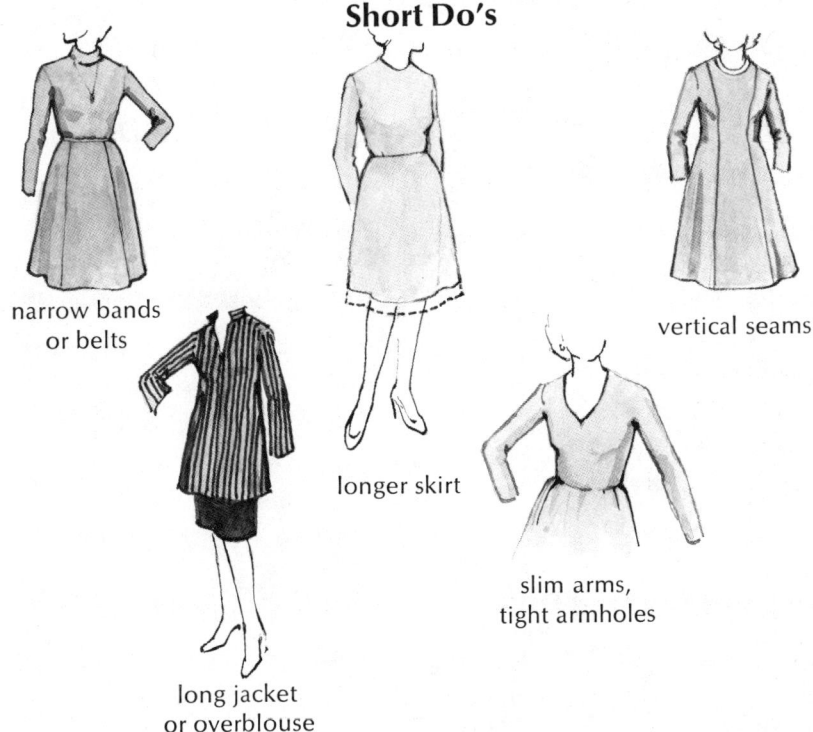

Short Don'ts

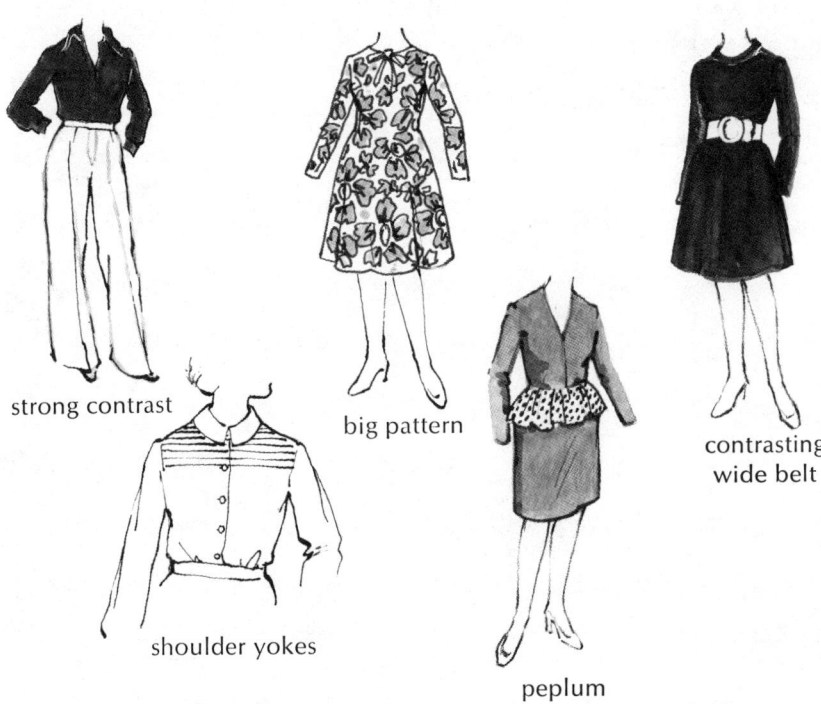

Long-Waisted Do's

Boleros
Vests
Wide belts in contrasting
  colors
Short jackets
Short overblouses
Darker tops
Horizontal stripes at the top
Wide waistbands

Long-Waisted Don'ts

Waistlines that ride 2" above
  your own
Narrow belts
Tucked in blouses and body-shirts
  without belts

Short-Waisted Do's

Narrow belts
Narrow waistbands or none on
  skirts and slacks
Overblouses
Empire waist
Bloused waistlines
Dropped waistline

Short-Waisted Don'ts

Wide belts
Waistlines that blouse, but
  should not

Long Waist Do's

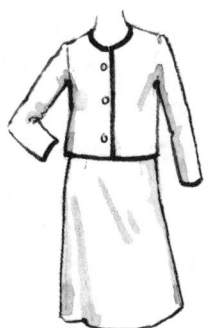
short jacket

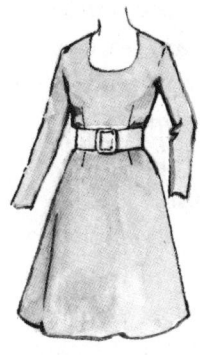
wide belt

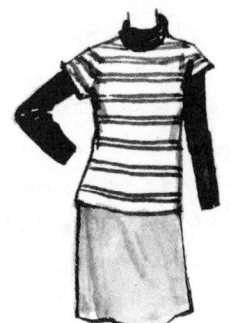
horizontal strip on top

Short Waist Do's

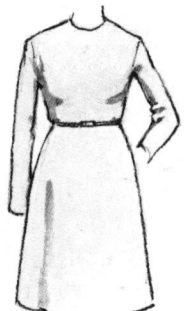
narrow belt, no contrast

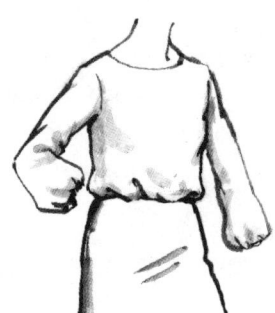
bloused waist

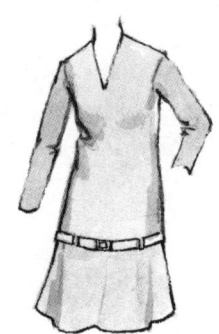
dropped waist

No Waist Do's

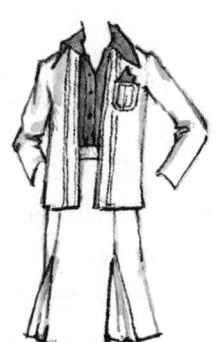
straight jacket falling below hip

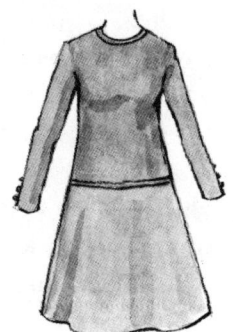
solid color

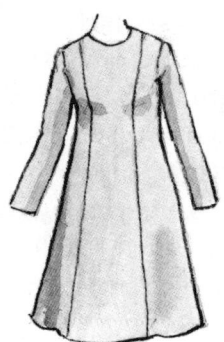
A-line

What we all want is the tall slim figure on which most clothes look best. Since that is not possible physically, what we are trying to do is make proportion and lines in our clothes create that illusion. If possible, go into the selling area in the store from the dressing room and see how the garment looks from a distance. This gives you the silhouette devoid of details to help you judge if you have lengthened and narrowed your figure.

If you are saying, "She did not mention my long legs, my short legs, my long neck, my short neck, my long arms, my short arms," I believe you have enough perspective here to help you work out your proportion problems. The right garment can help you camouflage anything wrong with your figure, and, believe me, most of us have something to hide.

YOUR FOUNDATION

Problems with your figure have not been ignored by you, I am sure. But some authorities in the foundation garment business accuse the average women of wearing what they please, instead of what they need. Let's see if you are wearing what you need.

Rule of Ten suggestions for a younger, thinner-looking figure:

1. Don't wear your bras or girdle too tight. You only look as though you were poured into a sausage skin.

2. Don't wear a short-line bra with a panty girdle if you are getting a roll at the waist. Get a long-line bra and hold it down with hooks, which fasten to the girdle.

3. To avoid the last problem, do wear a full-length garment. They are available in many choices of bra size and shape and stomach and buttocks holding quality. I am referring to the knit, pull-on, no-stays garments.

4. As you lose weight, which I hope you are doing, try to get rid of that stiff, full-length garment, which keeps you so rigid with its ironlike stays. Try one like I just mentioned and see how much freer

Big Shoulders

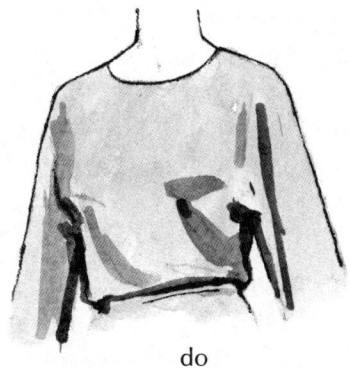
do

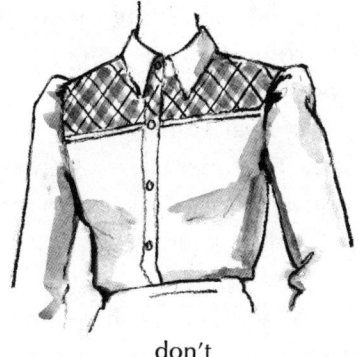
don't

Short Necks

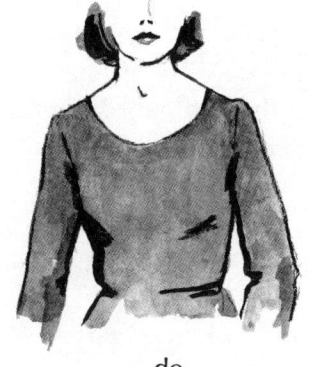
do

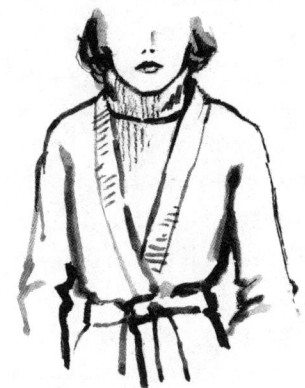
don't

Long Arms

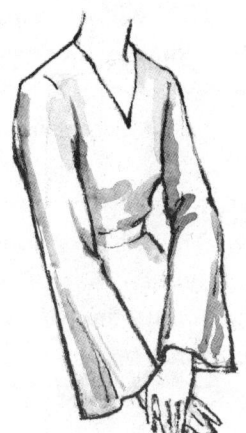
do

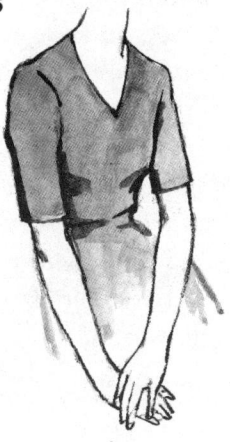
don't

you feel. Since I believe that stiff movement is more aging than most people realize, getting out of those stays is important. Look at the older women on the street, who look as though they are walking around in wooden boxes.

5. Do wear some kind of support if you have even a little excess weight. This seems like unnecessary advice for the over-corseted American woman but there may be those of you who started out with a girlish figure that needed no support, and the added weight or just skin sag has been ignored as the years slipped by.

6. If you are really heavy-busted, keep to fabric and not knits in your bras. The material that forms the cup should be light weight to mold to your form better. It should be cut on the bias and have no seam across the middle.

7. The padded bra is out and thank goodness. Remember the days of the molded, pointed, padded bras that gave everyone the same phony line? I hope you are not still wearing one.

8. Your posture can be affected by straps that are pulled too tight. Get the support you need from the bra itself. Not only that, but in lifting the garment they produce a roll along the top in back. The lower you can keep the line in back the more likely you are to avoid the roll. Please, if you have a roll anyway, stay away from tight-fitting tops.

9. There may be among you some who still may need garters. You can abandon them when you get rid of the stays. Panty hose are so much freer.

10. Know about the custom-made garments, which will be more costly than those you have been buying over the counter, but will help a problem figure. If you are big-busted and small-hipped, or big-hipped and small-busted, or have any variation of figure from the average, the manufactured garment may not exist that is right for you. Some department stores have their own custom departments. There are small custom shops in your community. There is a famous company named Berlé with a shop in New York, Neiman Marcus in Dallas, and the I. Magnim stores on the coast. Jeannette Sim of the New York Berlé was most helpful in advising me in this section.

ACCESSORIES

The accessories you wear and the way you wear them can be a very important and certainly inexpensive way to keep yourself up to date. Here are some do's and don't's that may alert you to the use of these decorative items in your wardrobe:

SCARVES

Size, shape, and material are fashion-dictated, like everything else, and can give you an "haute couture" look when worn with the latest knot or angle. Pick up an older dress, suit, sweater, or blouse with a scarf and it looks and feels like a new one. Scarves can hide the aging neck. They can hide the hair that needs attention. They can drape gracefully to give you elegance and drama or hug tight around the neck for warmth. Whatever their use, use them, but use them fashionably. When that long chiffon number you have always loved so much is out, lay it tenderly away.

BELTS

Belts are certainly a fashion item. The narrow tube tie belt, the chain belt, the self-belt, the wide flat belt, the wide buckle, the narrow buckle—they all have their day. With the purchase of a new belt, you can give a "this-year" look to more than one dress. Again, watch the store windows and fashion magazines for the trend and don't carry on with one that is dating your garment. I got a lot of mileage out of a beloved chain belt not too long ago, and I retired it with great reluctance. An interesting sidelight on that belt is that it belonged to my great-aunt, who wore it in the early part of this century.

GLOVES

Who has seen an opera-length glove since Queen Elizabeth's coronation? What has happened to the women's glove industry I wouldn't like to know, since gloves have been abandoned for decoration. The short white cotton glove with the summer dress or suit is still seen in good shopping sections of New York, but there are many more well-dressed women without them. I saw a die-hard recently who waved her beaded bag at me as her wheelchair pushed past. The hand holding the bag was encased in beautiful pink, embroidered doeskin. Shades of grandeur past! On her they were dear—you are too young. Save your gloves for winter, when a beautiful pair of suede gloves is still a joy.

HANDBAGS

Fashion arbiters speak of "the good bag" as the most telling part of your wardrobe. Sailing along in your Givenchy suit and a $5.95 handbag won't do. Paying good money for a bag can be amortized over a longer period of time than most other fashion items.

Of course you can keep the casual, inexpensive bag for the grocery shopping, and let it have a shoulder strap.

JEWELRY

Here is where you can really follow the fashion scene according to your purse strings. I hav bought more than one pair of earrings in the dime store. They may not stand up very long, but they'll last as long as the green dress I bought them for. Chunky bracelets, big or little opaque-colored beads, long chains are all available at small cost. If you can afford it, and you buy them in a good store when they first become popular, they will obviously look better—and cost more. However you do it, keep your jewelry current with the times.

Earrings

Wear them. No woman ever was accused of not caring what she looks like if she makes the effort to wear earrings—but wear them right. Whatever your facial structure or hairstyling, remember proportion. Huge button earrings on a big round face add to its width. Big round earrings on the small face overpower it. Just be aware of proportion and you will work it out. Just be aware, again.

It seems unnecessary to point out the use of the right earring for the right occasion and costume, but maybe not. I do see some of the strangest combinations as I walk along the street. I hope you stick to the tailored for the casual and save the sparkle for your long skirt.

Bracelets

Bracelets are feminine and dramatic. They can add color to your outfit and they can add elegance if you happen to have one made of diamonds. The only thing to watch is proportion, again. A heavy, thick bracelet on a thick, heavy arm is not pretty.

Rings

Rings have their fashion trends too. Currently, the young and dramatic are wearing them on every finger. Take a good look at your hands before you pick up this fad, you may not want to draw that much attention to them. I think we are in better taste to keep to good rings—in contrast to costume rings of fake stones and filled gold. However, if you have a collection of costume rings and they look good on your hands and are right with the outfit, wear them. I think I am only speaking personally here.

Pearls

It is a shame that pearls have to have their fashion, too. They are so flattering and their soft lustrous white picks up a dark garment so well. But the graduated pearls your husband gave you for your fifteenth anniversary will have to stay in the safety deposit box awhile longer. Pearl chokers are also a great loss. I wore them with everything, didn't you? They will be back in some form or another. in the meantime, be careful—they will date you.

Necklaces, Chains

Get out all of your long chains and beads. Small link chains, large link chains, multiple chains, all are *in* today—and out tomorrow. Just be quick to abandon them when they have been abandoned by fashion.

The only choker you are allowed is the new version: a stiff metal ring that springs open to hug the base of the neck, and sometimes has interesting pendants hanging from it or incorporated into it. They are very contemporary looking and smart.

Antique Jewelry

Antique jewelry is admirable, with reservations. The problem is using it in relation to the current fashions. It can be very dramatic, or it can be just old jewelry, which makes you look dowdy. Teenagers have taken up old jewelry and they get by with wearing inferior pieces, but on you and me it may just look old fashioned. So pick your best pieces, and wear them with care—and do consider having good stones put into contemporary settings. You will get a new thrill out of those old diamonds when you get them out of that old platinum filigree.

Before we leave jewelry, you should know the fashion rule that not more than three pieces of jewelry should be worn at one time, not including rings. And if your dress or suit has a multitude of metal buttons, eliminate one of these pieces.

The jewelry message is, obviously, keep alert and be quick to change, as in all the other accessories.

SHOES AND HOSE

SHOES

The fight between shoe styles and foot doctors will go on forever. The female foot has been crammed into foot-deforming shoe shapes through the centuries. Did you ever see a picture of Marie Antoinette's shoes? The toes of her satin and lace shoes could pick your teeth. There was an exhibit of costumes at the Metropolitan Museum that showed a shoe trunk, complete with twelve pairs of shoes belonging to a famous beauty of the 1920s. They could have belonged to Marie. Luckily, the casual and natural has been in fashion for some time, to the benefit and comfort of our feet. But—heels are getting higher and thinner as the skirts get longer, and I dread to think that these will ultimately dominate the scene. I have been too comfortable too long.

The human foot originally walked on grass, sand, and vegetation with give to it. The cement sidewalks of our city streets cause a jarring of the entire body with each step. Foot troubles develop. The first thought with the first problem is to head for the nearest drugstore. Too many people rely on these drugstore panaceas of plasters and spongy inner soles for too long. Problems develop that only an expert should handle. I am ashamed to say that I was two years late myself in going to a podiatrist. The agonies I could have saved myself, and the ugly shoes I bought that I don't have to wear any more. To wear fashionable shoes you have to take care of your feet.

Feet should be exercised, as we found in chapter 6. With diligent exercises our feet will be more supple, which will allow us to bend our feet at the instep for a springier walk. Shoes will fit better and we can adjust to a higher heel, if that is what we are going to have to do in the near future.

The number of women's shoes sold that fit improperly must far exceed those that are correct. Along with liking the style and color and heel height, there are fitting points to be considered. Does the instep fit snugly? Is the ball of your foot seated on the ball of the shoe? Is the counter too big or too small, making the shoe slip up and down at the heel or pinch severely for the duration of the shoe? Is the shoe too shallow, so that the upper side presses too hard against your toes? Is the shoe long enough and wide enough? Sometimes your feet change, and you keep on asking the clerk for a 6½A, when you should change to a 7B. (Some experts advise wearing a size larger shoe and wearing an inner sole to take up the slack.) Does the shoe have the right balance? Is your weight balanced back on the heel instead of thrust forward onto the ball of your foot? This is important for your posture, which, as you remember, is best with the weight on the heel. Also, podiatrists tell us that when your weight is on the back and moves along the outside of the foot to the toes in your walk you are saved a lot of foot troubles. Balance, I have discovered, is in the construction of the shoe and not in the height of the heel.

Fashion must be served through all of these fitting problems and sometimes it is not easy. If you find a style and last that is comfortable, you may buy the same shoe year after year, like the little lady and her hat. This easy solution does not allow for fashion changes—and your shoes are very much a part of your fashion wardrobe. Study your uniform shoes carefully and when they are out of fashion buy a new shoe with the same fit in all the right places but with a newer heel shape, a newer toe shape, a T-strap, a sling heel. Get a new lease on life with a new shoe. I told a friend the other day that I feel differently about myself when I wear certain shoes. I prance along in my open-toed sandals feeling sexy. My spirits are not raised with a low-heeled walking shoe. If shoes have a psychological effect on me, this must be true of a lot of women.

Depending on your location or life-style, or both, your shoe wardrobe will vary considerably. As in all other areas of fashion, no matter what your shoe needs are, the keynote is attention to detail. Even if you only wear slacks and the buckle loafer, changes of detail are there from year to year. The heel may be placed on the shoe at a different angle; it may be a covered heel or a leather heel; the tongue may be shorter or longer; or shaped a little differently. Notice details and care about them in all of your shoes. And, as in the rest of your wardrobe, the newer look will save you money by lasting longer fashion wise.

HOSE

If you have abandoned the hose that came in sizes for the "fits-all-sizes," don't. The subtle pressure of those constructed to stretch to your size are almost as bad for your feet as the pointed toe. This seems a simple enough choice to insure better feet. You can also help your circulation by wearing elasticized stockings. These are highly recommended if you are on your feet a lot or if you have circulatory problems, and they are not unsightly. (I knew a fashion shoe model who wore them in a very light shade on the runway—she covered them with sheer hose!)

If your legs don't look so young, due to surfacing blue veins, wear heavier hose. They don't have to be opaque or elasticized, just not the sheerest. And if they don't help enough, use a cover-up that you would buy at the cosmetic counter for facial blemishes. These noticeable problems, which speak of advancing years, are not pretty for others to look at and so easily can be camouflaged.

Watch that the shades of natural, suntan, taupe are the right tone for your outfit, and especially your shoes. I looked down in the broad daylight the other day and discovered my hose were far too brown a tone for the light beige shoes I was wearing. You can err also in the use of taupe shades. This greyed-up tan color should be saved for black, gray, and navy. Keep the suntans for white, brown, and most pastels. The most easily adaptable for all are the natural, or nude, called different names by different manufacturers. Black skin looks better in brown tones, which should be obvious, but I see a lot of light shades, which end up giving a grayish appearance to the legs.

Don't forget the knee-highs, which can be so comfortable under slacks.

HATS

When my eighty-five-year-old mother stopped wearing a hat to church, I knew the jig was up. Hats were out! Then why am I writing about them? Because there remain two types of die-hard hat wearers: those who feel that certain outfits are enhanced by the right hat and those who have always worn a hat—the same hat bought for summer, winter, fall and spring, same shape, different colors. The latter group I would like to discourage. I agree with the first group, and here are some of the shapes that are acceptable:

THE FUR HAT

The good fur hat, worn with an untrimmed coat, can be smashing. The fur hat that matches (really matches) a fur coat can be very dramatic. Fur hats are worth the investment, as they can be worn for a long time.

THE BERET

The beret is a simple shape, good with suits and coats if your hairstyle and face shape can handle it. The secret to wearing the beret is in the angle at which it is tilted. French women really know how to do it. No matter what size the collar or how high it rides on the neck, this shape never gets in the way. How many times have you bought a brimmed hat and spent the rest of the winter holding your head at an angle so the brim doesn't hit the collar?

THE TURBAN

The turban is a very dressy-style hat, which gives height to the short woman and is becoming to many different face shapes.

THE TAILORED FELT

It is hard to make an all-encompassing statement about these hats, because you may be an exception. What I really want to say, you see, is that these are for the younger woman. There are more sins of shape committed in this material than any other. The only rule I know is from observation. If that hat has such idiosyncracies of line in crown and brim that you look at the hat and not the face beneath, then it is wrong. Leave this hard material, which creates hard, strong lines, to those whose younger faces can enhance them. (This does not mean that a lovely white-haired woman couldn't wear a good shape in a great color and wow them.)

THE WIDE-BRIMMED STRAW

Be careful: There is something awfully "dowager" about this hat, if worn in the wrong place at the wrong time. If you are planning to wear that new pink beauty to the wedding, go ahead. Just make sure the crown is round and head-hugging, to give it as young a look as possible.

THE CLOCHE

This has returned from the flapper days, with variations. The short, uncurled hairstyling, which is currently with us makes a perfect roost for the cloche. Just pull it down, pull a little hair out at the sides, and away you go. Good for short women, as the crown is usually higher.

And if you don't want to wear a hat, don't. There are no longer any rules. Just remember that the wrong hat can age you faster than any other piece of clothing.

The famous French novelist, Colette, wrote a short story about an older woman who had a young lieutenant lover. He came to see her on every leave. Things went along very well until one day, as he was leaving, she playfully picked up his lieutenant's cap and put it on at a rakish angle. The romance did not survive the picture she presented.

SHOPPING

Rule of Ten suggestions for better shopping:

1. Shop early in the season, with your fashion knowledge firmly in mind. Shop in May for summer, February for spring, August for fall and winter. In the fashion business there is a term called "the first cutting." In subsequent orders of the same garment, there can be a reduction of effort and a substitution of materials. Shopping early insures you of a good selection of sizes. How many times have you found the very thing you can't do without and lo, your size has been sold out. Also, any fittings will be ready for you twice as fast as in midseason.

2. On the other hand, watch for sales that come at the end of the season. Keep your fashion awareness going strong on these shopping trips. The store of your choice may have some good buys, but you will have to know the style that is at the end of a trend, which won't carry you over into next year very fashionably. Sometimes it is fit. The shoulders are much too big for the rest of the garment, or the waist too small, or the bustline all wrong. I have found, more than once, that a size 10 hangs in all directions like a size 14. Someone in the marking room goofed three months earlier and cost the store a sale. But a sale item in a better dress that is right is a treasure. Many smart women do all their shopping this way.

One warning! Be sure the sale item that you want to buy is one you will have use for. If you get carried away in the shop, get home, and find you have no place to wear it, it's no bargain.

3. Plan ahead on your wardrobe, so you don't have to buy all your expensive items in the same season. This year you can buy a better coat, if you don't buy a suit until next year. I broke this rule, by necessity, one time with near disaster. I had a suitcase stolen, with all of my best clothes in it. Armed with the insurance money and confronted with a marvelous sale, I bought a winter suit and a winter coat. The next fall there was an attempt to drop the hemline to mid-calf, and both coat and suit barely covered the knee. Luckily, the fashion authorities came up with the theory that length was the individual's choice at this point and I was saved. I wore them both for five years.

4. Find a shop you like and a saleswoman you can trust and you can save yourself a lot of time and effort. The saleswoman can be in a small shop or a large store but she can be invaluable to you if you haven't the time or interest to study the details of current fashions. She will inform you of newly arrived merchandise, special purchases and markdowns. The warning here is not to get into a rut. Have ideas and some knowledge of your own, otherwise she might keep in mind the particular type of garment you like and you will go trotting to the store time after time, only to buy variations of the same garment—your uniform.

5. Shop alone. Some of my biggest wardrobe mistakes have been at the urging of a companion. "Oh, Dorothy, that is just divine. You simply have to buy it." Catastrophe! You can all recall similar experiences, I am sure. Someone else's taste cannot be yours and you find yourself carried away with flattery, knowing in your heart that you are doing the wrong thing.

6. Plan each seasons clothes ahead, so you aren't madly buying five pairs of shoes to match all of those colors you have just added to your wardrobe. If you pick a central color, your scarves and blouses and all your accessories will work together.

7. Buy what you can afford. Genevieve Antoine Darieux, in her book *Elegance*, speaks of amortizing your clothing purchases. It is, certainly, a good way to judge the cost of what you have bought. How many times have you worn it? The expression, "I didn't get much wear out of it," means that it was more costly than a much more expensive item, which you might have worn every day. Following this thought, it seems to lead to skimping, if your budget is limited, on the casual dress and spending more on the suit and coat.

8. Now, to contradict myself, let yourself go once in awhile and buy something on impulse. According to your income, it can be an accessory item or a coat you don't need but fell in love with. These loves usually amortize out very well, as you will reach for them many times.

9. Watch your posture as you stand before the mirror admiring your prospective purchase. Are you pulling in your stomach, pulling back your shoulders and standing in lovely graceful poses to show off the piece like a model? It may fit differently when you get it home and relax into your usual slump. You may find all kinds of faults with it and not even realize why. Hopefully, the slump is disappearing after your strenuous workout in chapter 6.

10. Consider your life-style and your community in your selection of clothes. If you always have dressed with great flamboyance, and you move in a social situation where this style makes you overdressed, be aware of it and conform. Keep your creative talents alive by wowing them at the dinner dance. On the other hand, if your clothes have been suburban housewife and your husband's change of business puts you into a more elaborate social whirl, conform. Social groups can be very cruel if you deviate too far from their standards of dress.

HAIR

No fashion picture would be complete without talking about your hair. Your crowning glory can become your downfall into the aging pit. The "this is the way I wear my hair" attitude will stop any change suggested by your hairdresser every time. Operators don't often take a chance and push a change. They can't afford to send you away from their shop a dissatisfied customer, passing the word that Adrian's Salon ruined your hair. If you have been taking other improvements seriously, you have to keep your fashion awareness going to include your hair. Next to complexion, hair is the second part of your appearance that people are first aware of, either consciously or unconsciously.

Here are some things to consider in dealing with your hair:

HAIRSTYLING

1. No. Hair hanging to the waist, unless you are on the island of Tahiti.

2. No. Shoulder length is far too girlish.

3. Maybe. A short ponytail at the neck can be comfortable at home or on the beach.

4. Yes. Not any longer than an inch and a half from the shoulder in back and pulled up to the crown from the sides. It can be held up with either a barrette or a velvet ribbon. This is especially good when the hair is quite white. It is particularly youthful, but requires plenty of hair on the sides. Since that is where the hair starts to thin, this styling will have to be ruled out by some.

5. Yes. Long or shoulder-length, long enough to pull back into a low knot or brush up into a knot at the crown. Be sure that this knot is high enough, because there is a half-way angle that is very Irish washwoman.

6. Yes. The French twist is severe but chic. It is especially good for the woman who is going to follow up with high-fashion clothes. It is good for the short neck, lifting the eye up. Here, as well as in the previous high knot, the trick is to brush the hair up from the sides to the top and not horizontally along the sides of the head. This is extremely important for the sleek look you are trying for. Prematurely white hair with the still young face can handle this styling very well. I like it with any age face, provided the bone structure is defined enough. If this is too severe for you, it can be softened with shorter curls or wisps around the face, or even full bangs.

7. Yes. Below the ear length all around. The actual length will depend on the styling and your face shape. It can be worn slightly turned under, pageboy style, or with a looser, softer curl, with or without backcombing at the crown. You may want to give the top a little lift, depending on the shape of your face. This styling will swing and blow and fit into the present freedom of dress. Swinging is sexy!

8. Maybe. For the boy cut you will have to have a very good hair-

Hair Styles

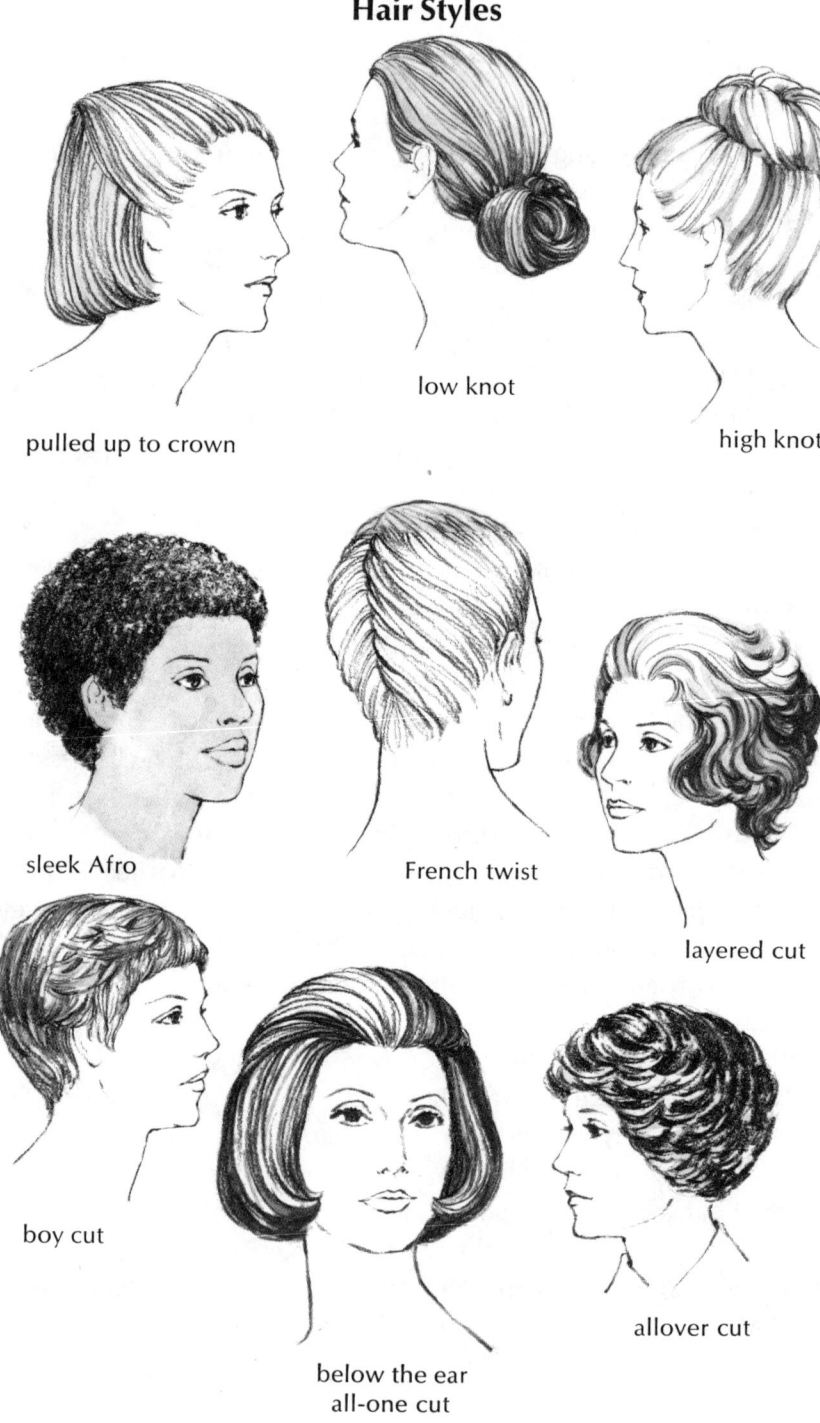

stylist give you a perfect cut, just for you. The shape of the face must be accounted for. For instance, it should be cut close to the sides of the head for the thin face or with more fullness to balance a full jaw. The naturally curly hair with all-over ringlets can be cute but surprisingly mannish. Since women lose some of their femininity as they get older, this whole type of cut must be watched with extreme care. I hope that if you are getting too mannish a look with it you will recognize that and not keep wearing it because it is so easy.

9. Yes. The Afro. A sleek Afro cut on the older black woman with white or graying hair is very smart. I don't see many on the street, so I suspect that this may be considered too young. I don't.

10. Yes. This is uniform and how can I decry it. This two- or three-inch length over the entire head with a curly permanent is on every head over fifty, and on many under that age. To enjoy the benefits and get some distinction, try some variations:

   a. Bangs, if your face can handle them. If you want to see how you look, pin them into place before you cut them and take a good look. I will never forget having my hair cut by a good friend one day (a mistake in the first place). Snip, snip, and I suddenly had bangs. "Well, that was a mistake." he said casually as he stepped back to view the results. It took six months of anguish before they grew out.
   b. Shorter hair, cut at the sides of the forehead, which can be either wispy or softly fluffy.
   c. Brush it out and let it blow. The day of the tight sausage curl is gone. It is all in the angle that the hair lies, not in the curl. Beware of hair that looks like a cap.
   d. Keep the back of the hair loose. I have seen terrible examples of lovely, fluffy, soft treatment around the face—then boom! it flattens out at the top and back, creating an ugly profile. Look at your hair in a hand mirror every time you get dressed, so you will see the whole picture.
   e. Make sure the fullnesses are in the right place for your whole facial structure.

11. Yes. The short layered look. Longer hair at back and sides and cut in a varying number of shorter layers. A real pro has to cut this one.

Figure problems to be considered in choosing your hairstyle:

1. The tall, thin woman must have a little fullness, or she will look like a pinhead.

2. The heavy-bosomed woman should have fullness to balance the heavy top. This woman can take a little more length if her neck is not too short.

3. The short-necked woman does well with the upswept hair or a very short cut.

4. The heavy-hipped woman needs some fullness to balance the hips.

5. The outsize-shouldered woman should wear longer and fuller hair.

6. The short woman should have some lift to her styling, especially at the crown. The day of the high, teased hair is gone, however, so the slight tease is all you are allowed. Even though the fashion for the highly teased, highly sprayed concoction has been frowned upon for some time, there are more than a few running around the streets. Don't you be one of them.

7. For everyone, regardless of stature, we are back to the proportion that is seen in silhouette.

YOUR HAIR COLOR

This is up to you. Kenneth, in his book, *Kenneth's Complete Book on Hair,* claims that half the women in the country color their hair and about half of those with gray hair are covering it as well. When you look at the available dyes, tints, and rinses on the shelves of the drug and department stores, you can believe it. Great strides have been made since the days of lifeless dyes, used by great-aunt Bertha, whose roots always seemed to show and no one was ever fooled by that dull color. That beautiful gloss, with lovely highlights right out of a bottle, which you can now get, makes it much easier for American women to enhance their appearance.

There are several choices you can make in dyeing your hair. You can use a dye that will wash out in a few weeks. (Read the label to see how long the dye lasts, as it varies.) There is a rinse that washes out with each washing. This gives the hair body, and it can still leave some gray showing. If you commit yourself to a full dye job, you must be prepared for periodic retouching at the roots for as long as your hair remains that color.

There are considerations to adding color to the graying hair. You can use an allover, one-color dye up to a certain age; but when it comes time to let some gray show through, it is wise to go to a good hairdresser. To avoid the hardening effect of solid color around your face, a competent operator will spend a great deal of time applying color to small strands. She will know the right color to use and will be able to judge where the color should be used. Why not let your hair go and let nature take its course? It may work for the blond, black, or redhead, but color can get very drab with brunettes. As the strands whiten, the original hair color waters down and you could look very mousey. The highlighting method keeps your hair a becoming shade, and the gray is there too.

If you are going to try streaking or highlighting at home, you had better have a competent friend help you. In the first place, you can't keep your arms up that long; and second, you can't control the size of the strands very well, especially in the back. Some kits have perforated caps to pull the strands that are to be colored through. You have probably observed the checkerboard pattern of some "loving care at home" jobs. It *can* be done well, but it requires patience. There is a new method that is done by painting the strands with a brush, which works very well on blond or light brown hair.

The graying blond can use very soft, very light dyes, which blend into the gray and are very soft around the face. Blond hair can be kept young-looking longer than other colors without looking artificial or hardening the face.

Black hair usually whitens faster. It is pretty, but as the gray starts to appear you may want to help it along by a trip to the hairdresser.

If you are one of the "as nature intended" in your group, you should know about rinses that bring out the white in your hair. These will brighten it a lot. They are also good for pure white hair, which tends to yellow. No lavender rinses, please.

WIGS

> The Golden hair that Galla wears
> Is hers: who would have thought it.
> She swears t'is hers—and truth she swears
> For I know where she bought it.
> —Sir John Harrington

The wig fad is pretty much out. The looser, shorter hair of the last few years is not so easily duplicated in a wig. Wigs had their day when the teased, sprayed hairstyles were with us and, also, the very long hair down the back. This does not mean that they do not have their uses. They are valuable if:

1. There has been an illness, the hair has thinned visibly, and the wig is needed to conceal this.

2. The hair is so fine that the collapse of a hairdo is predictable.

3. You are a model and you need quick hair changes. (This does not apply to many of us.)

4. You are traveling and you do not have time for a hairdresser or any home remedies. This is really important on a long trip, with many changes of locale. I know, because I tried it.

5. You are a dedicated swimmer and cannot possibly get your hair in shape for that dinner engagement.

6. You don't have time to wash your hair and it looks a little glum.

7. With the cost of hairdressing rising all the time, the use of a wig for the interim periods can save you a few hair appointments.

8. You have messed up your hair with bleaching and dyeing until it is almost beyond repair. You can give it a rest and time to grow out, with a wig to make you presentable for the duration.

You buy a wig according to your pocketbook. The first choice, at the top dollar, is European human hair, which can run anywhere from $300 to $600, custom made and styled for you. These are available only at wig boutiques around the country. Synthetic wigs come in a good variety of styles and colors and, with the price range from $25 to $60, they are by far the ones most generally bought. These are not the ones you see on tall racks out on the sidewalks on 14th Street in New York. $3.00 to $7.50? I am inclined to sneer as I spot them on a head a block away. But this is very snobbish—they must be a real godsend to the woman who cannot afford a beauty parlor and does not have much time; and they certainly keep her head warm in the winter.

Frank Ashton of the Enny of Italy wig salon in New York gave me some very good pointers on wigs: Watch the mesh to which the hair is attached. Try to get it as light in weight as possible. The handmade is the lightest, but some are a combination, the handmade being the closest to the face. The machine-made is the least costly and consequently heavier. For those of you who say, "I can't stand wigs, they are so heavy," this is good to know if you are dubious about buying a wig.

I brought up my favorite complaint about wigs being too thick and Mr. Ashton told me something I should have known long ago. Wigs can be thinned. They have to be done professionally by a good hairdresser but they can be improved considerably. The reason they are not made thinner in the first place is that there must be enough hair to cover the mesh base.

There are two methods for the construction of synthetic wigs. They can be made of fibers, which can be styled by a hairdresser to suit your desired changes, or baked in a style that lasts for life. It would seem that the former would be more desirable, but if your wig has to be styled each time it is washed, it could get quite annoying and costly. On the other hand, if you choose a style that is good on you and the only care you have is dousing it up and down in some suds occasionally, it does have its advantages.

The hairline of a wig must be covered, so watch very carefully the match to your own if you are going to comb your own hair over the hairline and incorporate it into the wig hair. For those of you who want a complete change from your own color, you will have to wear bangs well or get just the right wisps falling from the sides and front of the wig to frame your face. Keep in mind that these can be cut to suit you, so if you find a color you like and the hair around the face isn't becoming, you don't have to live with it.

HAIRPIECES

Hairpieces can be valuable assets and they come in enough colors to match your own hair fairly easily. They are either attached to a small comb that slides into the needed area, or they can be held in place with bobby pins. Think of them if:

1. Your hair is thinning and a cluster of hair in a strategic place can camouflage the problem.

2. You need a new hairdo to lift your spirits and you can play around with your hairpiece to create a new effect.

3. You are going to a Big Event and you want to get away from the old humdrum you, you can use the hairpiece to become an elegant creature.

In dealing with your hair, you may have noticed that I have avoided any advice on hair care. This is because statistics show that most women over fifty go to a hairdresser. If, by chance, you do not, the only advice I will give you is to wash it often. Wash it with a change of shampoos from time to time and use those marvelous rinses that give the hair body. Hair authorities say that you can wash your hair as often as you please. Shampooing does no harm to the hair if the soap is thoroughly rinsed out.

Bibliography

Carson, Bryta. *How You Look and Dress*. New York: McGraw-Hill, 1969.

Clairol. *Happy Healthy Hair*. New York: Popular Library, 1975.

Crenshaw, Mary Ann. *The Natural Way to Super Beauty*. New York: David McKay, 1974.

Dariaux, Genevieve Antoine. *Elegance*. New York: Doubleday, 1964.

Garland, Madge. *The Changing Form of Fashion*. New York: Praeger, 1970.

Heilman, Joan Rattner, ed. *Kenneth's Complete Book on Hair*. New York: Dell, 1974.

Horn, Marylin J. *The Second Skin*. Boston: Houghton Mifflin Co., 1968.

Kaszas, Joan. *Hair: Care for It and Keep It*. New York: Barnes & Noble, 1974.

"Reflections: How to Dress to Correct Spot Figure Problems." *Models Circle Magazine*. February 1976.

Tuit, Ann. *How to Fit Clothes*. New York: Drake, 1972.

Walker, Morton H. *Foot Health*. New York: Arco, 1972.

9
Summing Up

It would have been a waste of time if you had read this book without making any personal changes at all, now wouldn't it? I really do not think it is possible. Maybe you did nothing but buy a new lipstick. Maybe the time has not come for you to make a major move, like enrolling in a French class or losing thirty pounds. Maybe you won't use the fashion knowledge you have gained until you are standing in front of the mirror the next time you are in a fitting room. Whatever help this book has been or will be to you will be based on the attitude you brought to it, so there obviously will be varying results. My sincere hope is that it has planted many seeds in all of you.

Here are my top ten choices of changes that I feel will make you a healthier, younger-looking and younger-thinking woman for the rest of your life:

1. Attitude toward Yourself. These ten choices for your better future will not all be in order of importance, but this one is: the growth of your self-assurance. If this book has inspired you to acquire a new hairstyle, a more alert step, a thinner waist, or an absorbing outside interest that is great, because each change has added to your attitude toward yourself and to your inner strength. You have attained an alertness to changes that can create a better you, and through these changes you will develop increasing self-assurance.

2. Posture and Movement. For your visual effect on the world, your posture and movement are more important than the right hat. They reveal what you think of yourself: your self-assurance, the lift of the diaphragm, the forward step, the turn of the torso—all are youthful and therefore crucially important. Since I am allowing myself only one choice, I feel that the lifted diaphragm is the most visually important. Think of it constantly, and if you can think to pull your shoulders down at the same time you have it made. Every time you catch yourself drooping, pull up. Seated, you have the look of someone who is alert and interesting—and you lose years. Standing and walking, your whole body reacts. Your head pulls up, you step out with more assurance, and you are ready for the torso twist that releases you from the rigidity of movement so commonly displayed by the majority of your peers.

3. Facial Expressions. This one will surprise you, since I did not dwell on this in the text. However, in searching for these ten most important improvements, I found myself going back constantly to expressions. Watching friends, people on the street, people I work with, I became aware of the expressions that were detrimental to appearance and personality.

Facial expression comes from thoughts in your brain, which control the muscles in your face. Since your unconscious thought can make frown lines and pull down the corners of your mouth, let us reverse the procedure and think consciously of changing the frown lines and the mouth corners. Maybe, when you work with the muscles that create happier expressions, you can lift your spirits, too. Maybe, if you pull your forehead muscles back at the hairline when you burn the spinach, you won't ever be disturbed over having one less item for dinner.

The beautiful woman with the perfect makeup will have wasted a lot of time and money if she has an expression that reflects bitterness, anger, or self-pity. To be sure you are not guilty, too, catch your reflection in mirrors and store windows as you pass by. To cure any unpleasant expressions, work before a mirror, pulling your facial muscles until your look is happier. Exercise these muscles as described in chapter 2 and make yourself aware of the right muscles to pull whenever you feel a bad thought coming on. If you go about looking as though you could bite nails, why bother with the false eyelashes?

Don't forget that your eyebrows can create bad expressions. If they are too close together, they can give the effect of a frown. If they are drawn too far down at the ends, they give you a depressed look you may not feel at all.

4. Makeup. My choice for a successful makeup is a negative one. Today's fashion in makeup is the natural look. The worst errors are committed in using strong colors and strong lines. This effect literally shrieks "out of date." If the over-madeup woman thinks she is hiding her age beneath the paint, she is badly mistaken. There are cosmetic authorities who say that the older woman looks best with no makeup at all. I don't agree with that, because I know that flaws can be concealed and good facial points accentuated without showing any obvious makeup at all. I knew a girl at one time who worked in cosmetics. On her honeymoon, her husband said to her one morning, "I was almost afraid to marry you because I didn't know what I might find under your makeup. Now I know you are really beautiful." The girl smiled prettily, aware that at that moment she had on four different cosmetics.

5. Skin Care. Since we can't put that dermis layer of our skin back into its younger state, the best we can do is to preserve the epidermis: Use a moisturizer both day and night. "Moisturizer" has become the magic word in the cosmetic business and is often combined with lotions and creams designed for other purposes. Be sure you get one that is a true moisturizer. You will be rewarded with a skin smoother to the touch, and small lines will miraculously disappear. I can vouch for one miraculous disappearance. I visited a friend for two weeks not long ago, presenting her with a bottle of moisturizer when I arrived. By the time I left, I was amazed at the decrease of lines around her eyes. It is such a simple, nontime-consuming habit to get into—with such beautiful results. (P.S. I hope you also are cleansing your skin every night and morning.)

6. Diet. I hope you have taken chapter 4 on diet seriously. Not only for excess weight, but for health as well. I know that it is hard to change lifetime food habits, but change is what this book is all about.

The most important thing to watch in your diet, as your age increases, is the consumption of animal fat, because of its tendency to form obstructions in the arteries. If diet can control circulatory problems, then common sense demands that you make some changes. You can easily cut the fat from the meat on your plate; you can buy the less fatty meats, such as chicken (don't eat the skin), veal, lamb, or fish; foods like stews, soups, chili, and spaghetti sauces can be eaten less frequently. Fat in these foods can be decreased somewhat by refrigerating first, then removing the congealed fat on the surface before reheating.

You can make sure that your cooking and salad oils are polyunsaturated (also cold-pressed); you can see that your oleo is soft (not the stick variety), and that butter no longer graces your table. You have long since changed to skim milk, I am sure. It is very easy to get cottage cheese, other cheeses, and ice cream with a skim-milk base these days. Buy them in health! (P.S. I hope you are cutting down on your sugar consumption, too.)

7. Vitamins. Take vitamins seriously, they can extend your active life. Since I am giving only one choice in each category, I will have to pick a multiple vitamin for your daily consumption. But you will really have to study labels to get the one with the most variety and with the most micrograms, milligrams, grams, USP units or IU per vitamin. You can't find this in the cheapest brands. If you don't know where to start, make a list of the recommended dosages in chapter 4 and take it with you when you set out to buy your vitamins. Don't shortchange yourself and pick the first one you look at—really shop for the best.

Since vitamins are a matter of individual need, you may find, from the list of vitamins at the end of the vitamin chapter, one that has proved helpful in a health problem that concerns you. You may want to augment your multiple vitamin capsule. Most capsules do not contain lecithin, which is helpful to the circulatory system, so I add that to my own diet either in capsule or powdered form. In the winter, you might want to take another vitamin C tablet. I add a 400 mg panathenic acid tablet, due to a physical problem that I give it credit for curing. You have to find your own way in selecting the vitamins and minerals for your own best health, but if you have bought the best multiple vitamin you can find, you will have made a good start.

8. Fashion. Teach yourself fashion awareness—this is my choice of what I would like to have you get from this book for your future clothes selections. Train your eye to see the details in fashion changes, such as shoulders, sleeves, cuffs, belts, lapels, necklines, and so on. This will give you a subconscious feeling of rightness in the garment you are about to buy. Of course, you will keep these details within the bounds that your body structure demands. Don't go out and buy the latest full skirt if your hips are 48″. Knowing the current fashion trends will save you money. By investing in coming fashions instead of those that are already on the decline, you will extend the useful life of your purchases. Fashion requires more study than most women realize. If fashion has never been your forte, this really can be a project for you and, I hope, a rewarding one—a project that will not only improve your appearance but will add to your self-assurance.

9. Acquire a New Interest. You can remember things you have passed by lightly, things you knew you would like to get back to sometime. Now is the time. Buy the paints and canvas. Get catalogs of courses available. Buy yourself a piccolo. Maybe all you will need to lift you up will be a new health-food cookbook. Take on a project that is helpful to others in a charity, a church, or a hospital. The reason I chose this action for my ninth improvement is obvious: If you are looking gorgeous, with all the right clothes and makeup and the best health in the world, and you are still sitting in the same rocking chair, you have not extended yourself enough. There is no way of telling, until you have tried a new interest, how much it can spark you, can give you a new self-image.

10. Self-Awareness. I keep coming back to this characteristic, because it seems to be the key to so much in our lives: our personal relationships, our health, our interests, our appearance, our physical being. Why, this is the whole book! If you develop a strong Mr. Right to look over your shoulder and help you really see yourself in every aspect, this book will have been of great value to you.

YOUR TEST

You were not warned at the beginning of this book that the following test was coming, so you will be taking it without premeditation. But the results of your test, taken now, will not yet show a true record of improvements. Some of them will take more time to implement. Some will inspire a delayed-action response. So I recommend that you put this book in a convenient place and take the test again in six months. Then take it again in a year.

How many improvements have you made in each of these categories to date? Check boxes in each category in which you have improved:

1. MAKEUP

Base:
   COLOR CHANGE ☐ TEXTURE CHANGE ☐

Rouge:
   COLOR CHANGE ☐ PLACEMENT CHANGE ☐
   TYPE CHANGE ☐

Eye shadow:
   COLOR CHANGE ☐ EYE-SHAPE CORRECTION ☐

Lipstick:
   COLOR CHANGE ☐ LIP-SHAPE CORRECTION ☐

Eyebrow change:
- SHAPE ☐
- COLOR ☐

Contouring to minimize flaws:
- NOSE ☐
- CHIN ☐
- FOREHEAD ☐
- OTHER ☐

Shading to minimize wrinkles:
- FROWN LINES ☐
- MOUTH CORNERS ☐
- FOREHEAD GROOVES ☐
- NOSE-TO-MOUTH LINES ☐
- CROW'S FEET ☐

2. SKIN CARE

Cleansing:
- PURE SOAP ☐
- SIMPLE OILS OR CREAMS ☐
- RINSING WITH WATER SPLASHES ☐

Thinning:
- WITH A PEEL ☐
- WITH ABRASIVE CLOTH OR SPONGE ☐
- WITH ABRASIVE CREAM ☐

Lubricating:
- USE OF LIGHT, EASILY REMOVED OILS AND CREAMS ☐
- REDUCTION OF UNNECESSARY CREAMS ☐

Moisturizing:
- NIGHT: WITH HEAVY CREAM OR VASELINE ☐
- DAY: WITH LIGHT ABSORBING LOTION ☐

3. DIET (regardless of weight)

Fat reduction:
- CUTTING FAT FROM MEAT ☐
- SKIM MILK ☐
- LESS FAT MEATS ☐
- VEGETABLE OILS ☐

Sugar reduction:
- NO DESSERTS ☐
- DIET SOFT DRINKS ☐
- SLOWING DOWN ON DESSERTS ☐
- NO SUGAR IN COFFEE OR TEA— OR CUTTING DOWN ☐

Starch reduction:
    CUTTING DOWN ON POTATOES ☐   CUTTING DOWN ON PASTAS ☐
                                                    NO WHITE BREAD ☐

Leafy vegetable speed-up:
    MORE SALADS ☐   MORE COOKED LEAFY VEGETABLES ☐

More root and other vegetables:
    MORE IN SALADS ☐   TWO COOKED VEGETABLES A DAY ☐

Add proteins:
    WHEAT GERM TO MANY THINGS ☐   GRAINED BREADS ☐
    NUTS TO SALADS AND VEGETABLES ☐   LEGUMES INSTEAD OF POTATOES OR PASTAS ☐

4. VITAMINS

Do you take a multiple vitamin?
    YES ☐   NO ☐

Do you take a B-complex capsule?
    YES ☐   NO ☐

Do you take any additional vitamins?
    YES ☐   NO ☐

How many?
    NUMBER ☐   NONE ☐

5. EXERCISE

Head:
    TWO EXERCISES A DAY ☐   WRITE IN ☐
    ONE EXERCISE A DAY ☐

Shoulders:
- TWO EXERCISES A DAY ☐ WRITE IN ☐
- ONE EXERCISE A DAY ☐

Upper arms and chest:
- TWO EXERCISES A DAY ☐ WRITE IN ☐
- ONE EXERCISE A DAY ☐

Waist and abdomen:
- TWO EXERCISES A DAY ☐ WRITE IN ☐
- ONE EXERCISE A DAY ☐

Hips and thighs:
- TWO EXERCISES A DAY ☐ WRITE IN ☐
- ONE EXERCISE A DAY ☐

Legs and feet:
- TWO EXERCISES A DAY ☐ WRITE IN ☐
- ONE EXERCISE A DAY ☐

Exercise
In bed:
- EVERY DAY ☐ WRITE IN ☐
- TWICE A WEEK ☐

Bathtub or shower:
- EVERY DAY ☐ WRITE IN ☐
- TWICE A WEEK ☐

Walking exercise:
- TWO A DAY ☐ WRITE IN ☐
- ONE A DAY ☐

Isometric exercises (pushing against table):
- TWO A DAY ☐ WRITE IN ☐
- ONE A DAY ☐

Pick-up exercise (picking up things from the floor):
- TWO A DAY ☐ WRITE IN ☐
- ONE A DAY ☐

Exercises while talking on the phone:
- TWO A CALL ☐ WRITE IN ☐
- ONE A CALL ☐

6 EXERCISES FOR MOVEMENT

Posture:
   FIVE A DAY ☐ WRITE IN ☐
   THREE A DAY ☐

Torso Movement:
   THREE A DAY ☐ WRITE IN ☐
   ONE A DAY ☐

Have you made these improvements
Going downstairs:
   YES ☐ NO ☐

Going upstairs:
   YES ☐ NO ☐

Sitting down easily:
   YES ☐ NO ☐

Getting up easily:
   YES ☐ NO ☐

Getting down on the floor:
   YES ☐ NO ☐

Getting up from the floor:
   YES ☐ NO ☐

7. WALKING

Have you analyzed your walk:
   YES ☐ NO ☐

Have you worked on any improvements:
   YES ☐ NO ☐

Do you think about your walk while you are walking to use these improvements:
   YES ☐ NO ☐

8. HAVE YOU BECOME AWARE OF:

Your conversations:
   YES   ☐   NO   ☐

Any of your relationships:
   YES   ☐   NO   ☐

Your self-assurance, and bettered it:
   YES   ☐   NO   ☐

Have you broadened your interests:
   YES   ☐   NO   ☐

How many:
   NUMBER   ☐   NONE   ☐

Have you improved your attitude with humor:
   YES   ☐   NO   ☐

Have you been helpful to others:
     Individually:
   YES   ☐   NO   ☐

     In groups:
   YES   ☐   NO   ☐

Have you found any personality flaws and improved them:
   YES   ☐   NO   ☐

How many:
   NUMBER   ☐   NONE   ☐

Have you done anything about understanding your finances better:
   YES   ☐   NO   ☐

Have you entered into any new activities:
   YES   ☐   NO   ☐

How many:
   NUMBER   ☐   NONE   ☐

Have you taken a good look at your sexual relations and made any improvements:
YES ☐ NO ☐

How many:
NUMBER ☐ NONE ☐

9. FASHION

Have you studied any fashion magazines or shop windows to become aware of fashion trends:
YES ☐ NO ☐

Have you studied your figure and found improvements to help you buy better:
YES ☐ NO ☐

Have you become aware of accessories to keep fashionable:
YES ☐ NO ☐

How many:
NUMBER ☐ NONE ☐

Have you changed any shopping habits:
YES ☐ NO ☐

How many:
NUMBER ☐ NONE ☐

Have you considered more becoming color choices:
YES ☐ NO ☐

Have you made any changes in your hair:
Styling:
YES ☐ NO ☐

Color:
YES ☐ NO ☐

Remember to check these answers again in six months. You will be surprised at the improvements you have made.

Index

Abrasive creams, 26
Accessories, fashion, 143–146
Alcohol calories, 69–70
Alcoholics Anonymous, 13
Alexander Principle, 101
American Medical Association, 78, 93
Andochronic (fatty acid), 76
Antique jewelry, 146
Art of Looking Younger, The (Shelmire), 27
Ashton, Frank, 161
Aslan, Ana, 92
Astringents, 25–26
Attitudes, 3–21, 165–166
   conversation, 8–10
   financial situation, 13–14
   humor, 10–11
   keeping current, 7–8
   personality and, 11–13
   self-assurance, 6–7
   self-awareness, 3–6
   sex, 17–20
   toward new interests, 14–17
   toward others, 11

Baby oil, 25
Backache (Krause), 100
Basic foods, eating daily, 61–63
Bathtub exercise, 106

Bed, exercise in, 105–106
Belts, 143
Berets, 150
Bioflavenoids, 87
Biotin, 86
Blaming others, 12
Blemishes, removing, 30
Blood vessels, surfacing, 35
Bossiness, 12
Bracelets, 145
Breakfast, 60
Breakfast table exercise, 107
Bridge, game of, 17
Briller, Sara Welles, 64
Bringe, Frank J., 66
Brown spots, 30, 32
   makeup for, 39
Burke, Edmund, 4
Burns, Robert, 54

Calcium, 89
Calorie-counting booklet, 59
Calories, 67–70
   in cocktails, 69–70
   "empty," 67–68
Cantor, Alfred, 76–77
Carbohydrates, 57, 75–76
   cutting down on, 66–67
Cardiovascular diseases, 57

Case of Delicacy, The (Sterne), 10
Chains, jewelry, 146
Cheek muscle exercises, 29
Chemo-surgery, 31–32
Choline, 81
Church work, 16
Clark, Linda, 61
Cleansing cream, 25
Cleansing lotion, 25
Cleansing skin, 24
Cloche (hat), 151
Clothes, selecting, 129–142
   accessories, 143–146
   for big bosom, 133
   for big hips, 130–131
   for big shoulders, 141
   hats, 150–151
   for long arms, 141
   for long-waisted, 138–139
   shoes and hose, 147–150
   shopping for, 152–154
   for short, with big bust, big hip, no waistline, 136–137
   for short neck, 141
   for short-waisted, 138–139
   for small bosom, 132
   for small hips, 130–131
   suggestions for younger, thinner-looking figure, 140–142
   for tall thin with no hips, 134–135
   See also Fashion awareness
Cobalt, 90
Colette, 151
College, returning to, 15–16
Color:
   eyeshadow, 44–46
   fashion awareness, 127–129
   hair, 158–160
   lipstick, 52
   for makeup foundation, 39–40
   rouge, 49
Constant complaining, 12
Contraceptives, 20
Conversation attitudes, 8–10
Copper, 90
Crash diets, 65
Crewel work, 15
Crocheting, 15
Current events, keeping interested in, 7–8
Cyanocobalamin, 80

Davis, Adelle, 64, 68, 79, 85, 88
Depilatories, 31
Dermabrasion, 31–32
Dermis (skin layer), 27–28, 32
Diabetes, 57, 75
Diet, 55–71, 168
   consulting doctor for, 70
   decision for, 58
   desirable weight (ages 25 and over), 56
   skin care and, 35
   ten "dont's" of, 66–70
   ten "do's" of, 59–66
   test for, 171–172
Diet formulas, 69
Diet pills, 69
Diet for a Small Planet (Lappe), 74
Diet Watcher's Gourmet Cookbook, The (Gold and Briller), 64
Dr. Cantor's Longevity Diet, 76–77
Dorian, Niles, 30–31
Dry skin, 24
Dyeing hair, 158–160

Earrings, 145
Ebon, Martin, 79
Enny of Italy (wig salon), 161
Epidermis (skin layer), 27–28, 32
Esoterica, 30
Ewald, Ellen Buckman, 64
Exercise, 99–109
   based on daily living, 105–108
   in bathtub, 106
   in bed, 105–106
   at breakfast table, 107
   for cheek muscles, 29
   for dieting, 59
   for eye sag, 29–30
   facial, 28–30
   frown, 28–29
   head and shoulder, 102
   hips and thigh, 103, 104–105
   legs and feet, 103, 105
   neck and shoulder, 104
   picking up, 107–108
   in the shower, 106–107
   telephone talking, 108
   test for, 172
   upper arms and chest, 102, 104
   waist and abdomen, 102–103
   waist and stomach, 104
   waiting in line, 106
   walking around the house, 106
   watching TV, 107
   See also Posture and movement
Eye sag, exercise for, 29–30
Eyebrows, making up, 41–44
   common structural faults and, 42
   pet peeves and, 44, 45
Eyelashes, false, 48

Eyeliner, 46–48
Eyeshadow, 44–46
   shape of eye and, 46, 47

Face-lifting, 32
Facial care. *See* Skin care
Facial expressions, 166–167
False eyelashes, 48
Fashion awareness, 121–163, 169
   accessories, 143–146
   color selection, 127–129
   development of, 121–123
   hair, 154–162
   hats, 150–151
   neckline, 123–124
   selecting clothes for your figure, 129–142
   shoes and hose, 147–150
   shopping for, 152–154
   shoulders, 124
   skirt length, 125
   sleeve treatment, 124–125
   test for, 176
   waistline, 124
   See also Clothes, selecting
Fats, 76–77
Fatty meats, 67
Finances, attitude toward, 13–14
Folic acid, 81–82
Food and Drug Administration, 32, 78, 89
Foods:
   dieting and buying, 59
   "empty" calorie, 67–68
   protein, 75
   using as a reward, 63–64
   vitamin A, 78
   vitamin B, 82
Ford, Eileen, 64
Fresheners, 25
Frown exercises, 28–29
Fur hats, 150

Gerraud, Don, 68
Gloves, 144
Gold, Ann, 64
Golf, 17
Gomez, Joan, 56
Gray hair, dyeing, 158–160
Guilt, feelings of, 12
Guitar, learning to play, 14

Hair, 154–162
   color, 158–160
   excess, removing or bleaching, 30–31
   in nostrils, 31

   styling, 155–158
   wigs, 160–162
Hairpieces, 162
Handbags, 144
Harrington, Sir John, 160
Hats, 150–151
Hauser, Gaylord, 64
Head and shoulder exercise, 102
"Hide it" sticks, 41
Hips and thigh exercise, 103, 104–105
Home decorating, 14–15
Hose, 149–150
Hospital volunteer work, 16
How Not to Die Young (Gomez), 56
H-3 (youth pill), 92
Humidifiers, 33–34
Humor, 10–11

Impotency, 19–20
Indelible lipstick, 51
Inositol, 81
Insulin, 75
Iodine, 89
Iron, 87–88

Jewelry, 144
Johnson, Norman, 121

Kane, Jean, 48
Kenneth's Complete Book on Hair, 158
Kettering, Charles, 37
Knitting, 15
Krause, Hans, 100

Lappe, Frances Moore, 74
Laughter, 10–11
Lecithin, 91
Legs and feet exercise, 103, 105
Let's Cook It Right (Davis), 64
Let's Get Well (Davis), 88
Light, for makeup, 38–39
Lind, James, 77
Lines, covering up, 41
Linolenic (fatty acid), 76
Lioleic (fatty acid), 76
Lip gloss, 51
Lipstick, 51–52
Lipstick brush, 51
Liver spots (brown spots), 30, 32, 39

Magnesium, 88
Magnifying mirror, 38
Makeup, 37–54, 167
   base (foundation), 39–41
   corrective, 52–54
   covering lines, 41

Makeup (*Cont.*)
   eyebrows, 41–44
   eyelashes, false, 48
   eyeliner, 46–48
   eyeshadow, 44–46
   lipstick, 51–52
   mascara, 48
   in proper light, 38–39
   rouge, 49–50
   test for, 170–171
   use of, 37–38
Male sexual capacity, 19–20
Manganese, 90
Mascara, 48
Masks, wrinkle, 34
Masters and Johnson, 19
Meals, planning ahead, 64
Meat, eating without folderols, 63
Mendelson, Irving, 99
Menopause, 18, 20
Metabolism, 65
Mirror, Mirror, on the Wall (Hauser), 64
Moisterizer, 24, 25, 33
   for facial, 27–28
   and makeup, 39
More Beautiful You in 21 Days, A (Ford), 64
Music, 14
My Secrets of Natural Beauty (Thomas), 35–36

Neck and shoulder exercise, 104
Necklaces, 146
Neckline fashion, 123–124
Needlepoint, 15
Neutrogena (skin soap), 24
New games, learning, 16–17
New interests, acquiring, 14–17, 169–170
Niacin, 80
Nostril hair, 31
Nutrition Against Disease (Williams), 75

Oil painting, 14
Oily/dry skin, 24
Oily skin, 24
Olmstead, Alan H., 13
One Bowl (Gerraud), 68
Other people, attitude toward, 11
Overindulgence, 12–13

Paige, Satchel, 99
Pantothenic acid, 80
Para aminobenzoic acid (PABA), 33, 82
Pauling, Linus, 84–85
Pearls, 145–146

Pencil outliner (lipstick), 51
Perfectionism, 12
Personality characteristics, self-awareness and, 11–13
Piano, learning to play, 14
Picking up exercise, 107–108
Pill, the, 20
Plants, growing, 16
Political volunteer work, 17
Pope, Alexander, 36
Posture and movement, 111–119, 166
   to rejuvenate muscles and regain younger movements, 114–115
   rule of ten for, 112–113
   test for, 174
   walking and, 115–119
   watching others, 119
   young movement for, 113–114
   See also Exercise
Potassium, 88
Proda, Betriz-Marie, 64
Protein:
   eating, 59
   food, 75
   need for, 74–75
Psychocybernetics, 7
Pyridoxine, 81

"Rape of the Lock, The" (Pope), 36
Recipes for a Small Planet (Ewald), 64
Red spots, 33
Regenerson shots, 92
Regression, 12
Riboflavin, 79
Rings, wearing, 145
Rinsing skin, 24–25
Rouge, face shape and, 49–50

Salad oil (to remove skin dirt), 25
Salicylates, 33
Salt and water retention, 67
Scarves, 143
Sebaceous glands, 32
Self-assurance, 6–7
Self-awareness, 3–6, 170
   test for, 175–176
Self-effacement, 12
Self-esteem, 6
Self-pity, 11–12
Selium, 90
Sewing, 15
Sex attitudes, 17–20
Shelmire, Bedford, Jr., 27
Shoes and shoe styles, 147–149
Shopping, suggestions for, 152–154

Shoulder fashion awareness, 124
Shower exercise, 106–107
Shute, Evan, 82–83
Shute, Wilfred, 83, 84
Silicone injections, 32
Skin care, 23–36, 167–168
   "don'ts" of, 32–36
   "do's" of, 24–32
   fancy ingredient items, 35–36
   sudden irritation and, 35
   test for, 171
   vitamins that affect, 34–35
Skin type, 24
   new product and, 35
Skirt length, 125
Skirt shape, 125–127
Slacks, 126
Sleeve treatment, 124–125
Slowing Down the Aging Process (Kugler), 91
Snacks, 68
Soap and water, 24–25
Starch, cutting down on, 66–67
Stay Young Longer (Clark), 61
Sterne, Lawrence, 10
Subcutaneous (skin layer), 27–28
Sugar, 75–76
   cutting down on, 66-67
Sulfur amino acids, 90–91
Sun exposure, 32–33
Sunburn, 33
Swimming, 17

Telephone-talking exercise, 108
Tennis, 17
Texture, makeup base, 40–41
Thiamine, 79
Think Yourself Thin (Bringe), 66
Thinning, facial, 26–27
Thomas, Virginia Castleton, 35–36
Threshold (Olmstead), 13
"To a Louse" (Burns), 54
Toning, facial, 25–26
Trace minerals, 90
Troisgros, Jean Baptiste, 17
Turbans, 150
TV-watching exercise, 107
200 Really Great Natural Food Recipes (Proda), 64

U.S. Department of Health, Education and Welfare, 74

Upper arms and chest exercise, 102, 104

Vegetables, eating without folderols, 63
Violin, learning to play, 14
Vitamin A, 77–78
Vitamin B, 78–82
Vitamin B-1, 79
Vitamin B-2, 79
Vitamin B-3, 80
Vitamin B-6, 81
Vitamin B-12, 80
Vitamin C, 84–85
Vitamin C and the Common Cold (Pauling), 84–85
Vitamin D, 85–86
Vitamin E, 82–84
Vitamin E for Ailing and Healthy Hearts (Shute), 84
Vitamin H, 86
Vitamin K, 86
Vitamin P, 87
Vitamins and minerals, 73–98, 168–169
   body requirements, 74–77
   life-span and, 91–92
   possible help from, 93–97
   for skin care, 34–35
   test for, 172
   See also names of vitamins and minerals
Volunteer work, 11, 16

Waist and abdomen exercise, 102–103
Waist and stomach exercise, 104
Waistline fashion awareness, 124
Waiting-in-line exercise, 106
Walking (around the house) exercise, 106
Walking and posture, 115–119
   correcting problems, 117–118
   test for, 174
Waxing process, 31
Weight, losing (too fast), 35
Which Vitamins Do You Need (Ebon), 79
Wide-brimmed straw hats, 151
Wigs, 160–162
Williams, Roger, 75
Women's Lib, 20
Wrinkle masks, 34

Yoga, 101

Zinc, 90